Praise for *Please eat...*

"*Please eat...* is an essential read for anyone trying to understand more about eating disorders in teenage boys. Bev Mattocks describes the story of her son's anorexia but also provides insight for other families facing this complex illness in a world where anorexia is still associated with teenage girls. Totally recommended." **- Sam Thomas, Founder of *Men Get Eating Disorders Too***

"Bev Mattocks shares her painful personal story so beautifully that the reader feels a deep connection. She models the tenacity needed by parents to stand up to these deadly illnesses for the long haul. This is a powerful account which health care providers around the world need to read before meeting with their first eating disorders patient." **- Becky Henry, Founder of Hope Network, LLC & Award Winning Author of *Just Tell Her To Stop: Family Stories of Eating Disorders***

"The world is slowly coming to realise that 'Boys Get Anorexia Too'. Bev Mattocks writes honestly and from the heart about helping her teenage son to overcome anorexia. Like ours, this is another success story of a family working together with friends, school and clinicians to beat this insidious illness. Many families will find great comfort from reading this story as well as much needed energy to fight the eating disorder." **- Jenny Langley, Author of *Boys Get Anorexia Too***

"This is a wonderful book. It's quite hard to read because the story is so painful, but easy to read because of the clarity and simplicity of style." **- Gill Todd, RMN MSc, former Clinical Nurse Leader at the Gerald Russell Eating Disorders Unit, Bethlem & Maudsley Hospitals, London**

"*Please eat...* is gut wrenching and touching. It captivated me and I could hardly breathe as I was reading it. I read the first six chapters in one sitting. Bev Mattocks has done such a great job of bringing her story to us in a vivid and personal way." **- Parent**

"Cancel your plans for the day when you open this book: the riveting story will have you caring and cheering for a family that the world needs to meet. If only the world knew the truth told in this memoir!" **- Laura Collins, Founder of *FEAST* (Families Empowered and Supporting Treatment of Eating Disorders) & Author of *Eating With Your Anorexic***

"Bev Mattocks is doing such amazing work empowering other parents and helping to raise awareness that boys get eating disorders too." **- Leah Dean, Executive Director, *FEAST* (Families Empowered and Supporting Treatment of Eating Disorders)**

"This book takes you on an emotional journey through the everyday reality of dealing with anorexia. If you're a health professional, read it to understand what parents are struggling with at home. If your friends or relatives think that anorexia is simply a refusal to eat, get them to read Ben's story. And if you believe anorexia is a girl thing, this book will sweep away your misconceptions." **- Eva Musby, Parent and Writer**

"*Please eat…* made me very emotional, it's hard recalling those moments when you realise that something is wrong. I am sure the book will be a valuable resource for many parents battling with eating disorders." **- Parent**

"When I first came across Bev Mattocks' story I was in the depths of despair with my daughter's anorexia which was spiralling out of control. Bev helped me realise that we were not alone, that we could help our daughter to recover and that, as her parents, we were part of solution and not the cause of her eating disorder. This is an empowering book." **- Parent**

"*Please eat…* is moving and engaging. Bev Mattocks creates a totally convincing picture of what it is like, and it's always respectful of her son. It certainly educates, so that a parent who's in doubt would recognise the symptoms. It reminded me of how confusing it can be, at the earlier stages, when the restricting is variable: just when you think your child isn't eating, suddenly they are… but you don't realise that it's because they think they've 'earned it' through exercise." **- Parent**

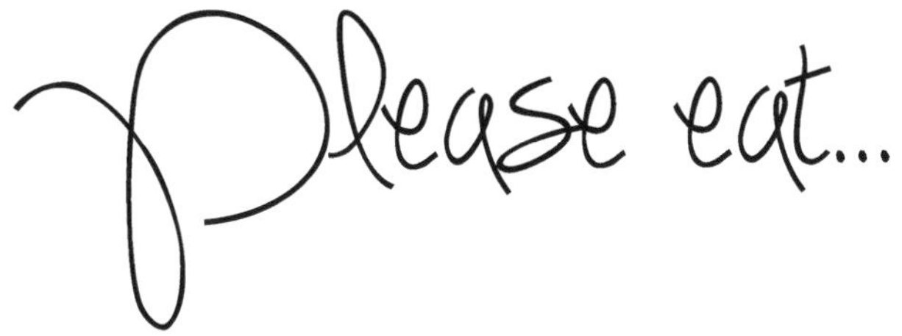

Please eat...

A mother's struggle to free her teenage son from anorexia

Bev Mattocks

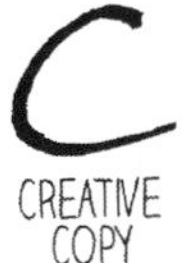

First published by Creative Copy 2013

www.creativecopy.co.uk

A catalogue record of this book is available from the British Library

ISBN 978-0-9575118-0-4

This book is a true story written from a personal perspective. Therefore it might differ from someone else's perspective of the same events. However, to the author's recollection, all events described here did take place. To protect identities and respect confidentiality, most names have been changed. Any resemblance of these names to actual persons, living or dead, events, or locales is entirely coincidental. Please note: this book is written as a source of information only and is not meant to be used, nor should it ever be used, to diagnose or treat eating disorders or other medical conditions. For diagnosis or treatment of eating disorders or other medical problems, please consult your own physician. The publisher and author are not responsible for any specific health needs that may require medical supervision and are not liable for any damages or negative consequences from any treatment, action, application or preparation, to any person reading or following the information in this book.

Find out more about Bev Mattocks at

www.anorexiaboy.co.uk

anorexiaboyrecovery.blogspot.co.uk

www.bevmattocks.co.uk

dedication

This book is for my dear friend, Sue. Thank you for always being there for us despite your own life struggles. You are an angel in the truest sense.

This book is also dedicated to my wonderful son - a young man of remarkable courage, determination and strength.

about the author

BEV MATTOCKS lives in the north of England with her husband and son, and works as a freelance advertising copywriter. She is a member of FEAST (Families Empowered and Supporting Treatment of Eating Disorders) and writes a popular blog about her experiences of supporting her teenage son through anorexia.

For more information, visit **www.anorexiaboy.co.uk**, **anorexiaboyrecovery.blogspot.co.uk** and **www.bevmattocks.co.uk**

author's note

BRIGHT, POPULAR AND A STAR on the rugby pitch, 15 year old Ben had everything he could want. But then, inexplicably, our food-loving teenage son began to systematically starve himself. At the same time his urge to exercise went extreme. In a matter of months Ben lost one quarter of his bodyweight as he plunged into anorexia nervosa.

But back in the summer of 2009 when Ben began to show classic signs of the illness, I had no idea that boys got eating disorders. As a result I didn't recognise the warning signs. I knew something was wrong and that it appeared to be getting worse, but I had no idea what "it" was. As the parent of a teenage boy you don't expect your child to get anorexia. You don't even think about it.

Please eat... A mother's struggle to free her teenage son from anorexia is my account of how anorexia crept into our normal, happy family life completely undetected. This book describes how, once we realised what we were dealing with, my husband Paul and I watched helplessly as the illness threatened to destroy our son on more than one occasion.

As a parent, I know how terrifying it is to discover that your child has a potentially life-threatening illness - and to discover that it's been developing undetected for months, maybe even years. I know what it's like to feel isolated, helpless and totally clueless about an illness that has the highest mortality rate of any mental health disorder. And

I know what it's like to have to wait months for treatment while your child fades away in front of your eyes.

When I sat down to write *Please eat…* I was acutely aware that I wanted to do my bit to help other parents and carers - not only to identify the warning signs of anorexia in boys but to show that there is a light at the end of the tunnel, and to describe how we got there.

I also wanted to highlight the importance of early intervention and effective treatment for young people with eating disorders, male or female, not just in the UK but wherever you live.

This isn't a story of despair. *Please eat…* describes how, with our help and through his own determination, Ben slowly began to recover from anorexia and re-build his life.

My son, Ben, has always been one hundred per cent behind this book. He is always nagging at me to "do more" to help raise awareness of eating disorders in a society where the illness is often shrouded in secrecy, shame and misunderstanding - and where there is still too little awareness of eating disorders in teenage boys. He has read through this book and made valuable contributions of his own which are included within its pages.

Even if we help just one family overcome this devastating illness by sharing our experiences then we have done our job.

Bev Mattocks, February 2013

important note

THIS ACCOUNT IS BASED ON a combination of memories, journal notes, blog entries, forum posts and other material which I compiled during the period that my son, Ben, was suffering from anorexia, and the years that led up to his illness.

It is important to bear in mind that everything described in this book is my own personal recollection of events and the emotions I was feeling at the time. It is the sole expression and opinion of its author. Other people's opinions, observations, memories, expression and recollections of the same events may differ. However, as far as I can recollect, allowing for the natural fallibility of memory, all the events depicted here took place as described.

Writing about someone else's life, especially your child's life, is very different from writing about yourself. It needs to be approached with respect, compassion and sensitivity. When people ask what Ben thinks about this book, I explain that he has always been completely behind me. He is as keen as I am to raise awareness of eating disorders in boys and help other families that might be facing a similar situation. However, to protect his privacy, I have given my son a false name. Most of the other names used in this book are false, too.

Over the summer of 2012 as I was putting this manuscript together, Ben and I went through it with a tooth-comb. He made his own comments and observations, many of which have been incorporated into this book. As with my own memories, one has to allow for impurities. But, to the best of our knowledge, this book tells our story, as it happened and in the way it happened.

Of course I am neither a clinician nor an expert; I am just an ordinary mum writing about the day to day experiences of living with a teenage boy recovering from anorexia.

As a result, the information provided in this book is not meant to be used, nor should it ever be used, to diagnose or treat anorexia, bulimia, EDNOS or any other eating disorder or medical condition. For diagnosis or treatment of anorexia, bulimia, EDNOS or any other eating disorder or medical problem, please consult your own physician.

Please note: the author does not endorse any specific eating disorder treatment approach or model. Each individual is different and the strategies used and outlined in this book may not be suitable for other families. Also, any references are provided for information purposes only and do not constitute endorsement of any websites or other resources. Readers should also be aware that the websites and other resources listed at the end of this book may change.

1

wired up to machines

IT'S THE 26TH JANUARY 2010, six months after 16 year old Ben's anorexia first began to emerge. I'm staring at the PC screen in the back bedroom of my house where I work as a freelance copywriter. Or, to be more accurate, where I am fighting a losing battle to keep my business afloat while my only child hurtles downhill to goodness only knows where.

This brief period - the hour or so between dropping Ben off at the school bus stop and the first frantic text I get as he struggles with another day at school - is the only time I really get to myself. But it's not as if I can switch off. Usually I'm reeling from the latest anorexia-fuelled meltdown in the fight to get Ben to school. More often than not I have my head in my hands, tears streaming down my face, hands fumbling for the tissues, wondering for the millionth time when - or even if - this nightmare will end.

By 9.30am I'm already jittery (these days I even take the phone into the bathroom with me). I can expect the first text around 9.30am. Sometimes it's even earlier. And sometimes it isn't Ben who gets in touch first but Sheila, the school nurse, concerned about the latest crisis Ben's got himself into.

Like the day I leave an over-distraught Ben at the bus stop but he fails to turn up for registration. Sheila calls to ask if he's made his way back home because "no-one remembers seeing him on the bus" and he isn't answering his mobile. My blood freezes as I search for my car keys, visions of driving up and down every single street in the city searching for Ben whose behaviour has become terrifyingly erratic. But Sheila calls back to say it's okay; they've found him crouching beneath a stairwell in the science block, sobbing his heart out. She's got him in the medical centre and is attempting to calm him down. I breathe a sigh of relief.

Or the time Ben suddenly downs his knife and fork, leaves his plate of food untouched and strides out of the school canteen unable to face eating lunch with his friends. The Head of Year charges after him and intercepts him en route to the river at the foot of the playing fields. A distraught Ben is returned to the safety of the medical centre where he spends the next hour or so talking with Sheila while I make my way into school to pick him up.

Sometimes it's a frantic three-way communication between Ben, Sheila and me. First Ben texts me from where he's barricaded himself in the boys' toilets like a frightened rabbit. I phone Sheila who attempts to entice Ben out. She calls me to say Ben's calmed down and is resting in the medical centre. Or, more likely, he's in a terrible state. Maybe it would be better if I took him home?

Or it might be a text from Ben who can't stop fretting about something I've planned for our evening meal. *The burger's far too fatty... Do you know how much fat there is in coconut milk...?* Worries like this can dominate the whole day until they explode into a mass of screaming, swearing, head bashing and the sound that never fails to chill me to the bone: a low pitched wail, like a wild animal in pain. Or the voice I've come to refer to as "the demon" - the voice of anorexia - the voice that isn't Ben's but which he uses whenever the anorexia is in control. It's slow, chillingly low and completely monotone. It's a voice I'd never heard before Ben succumbed to anorexia and I pray I will never hear again.

Today it's Sheila who contacts me first. Ben's with her in the medical centre. He doesn't look well. His heart is beating at around half the rate it's supposed to and his pulse is uneven. She'd like the hospital to see him.

I grab my car keys and rush into school. Ben's waiting for me in the car park. Sideways on I'm painfully aware that there's nothing of him: straight up and down, without any definition - a million light years away from the shapely calves and rugby playing thighs of just 12 months before. *Remember when we used to joke that Ben was made from concrete?* Ben hasn't played rugby since October. If he played rugby now he'd snap in half.

He turns round to face the car and I can't bear to look at the dark rings around his eyes set into the skull that looks far too big for his frail body. He climbs into the car silently, staring at the floor, his face expressionless. No greeting, no conversation. The anorexia has sucked every happy, positive emotion from his soul. He is completely numb.

And when he isn't numb, he's threatening to end his life or run away.

I put my foot down and drive the silent Ben towards the hospital on the eastern side of the city. One mention of "heart problems" and "pulse rate of 29" and we're spirited past the usual hospital queue. In a flash Ben's lying on a trolley and being hooked up to an ECG machine. Medical people are striding to and fro, checking the screen. I'm analysing their body language for clues because I can't read the expressions on their faces.

A doctor walks up to me with a clipboard. *Is there any history of heart problems in the family?* Er, my great grandma died of a heart attack back in 1917, does this count? *Is there anything else that might have sparked this off? Sport, maybe?* Well, yes, Ben's very sporty… *Aha, that makes sense. Athletes' hearts tend to be so fit and fine-tuned that the pulse rate can slow right down.*

Well, yes, for the past six months or so Ben has been doing some kind of high-intensity sport or exercise every single day of the week, usually several times a day. So I guess in a bizarre way you could say he is an athlete. But, as I tell the doctor, Ben has anorexia. He's had it for the past six months. Or at least that's when the signs of the illness first began to show. All this exercise, together with a massive reduction in food intake, is the reason why he's lost one quarter of his body weight since then. My gut instinct tells me that it's the anorexia that's brought us here, not the fact that Ben is a budding Olympian. His waif-like body looks virtually devoid of muscle these days, and isn't the heart a muscle?

The doctor writes something down and then takes some needles out of their sterilised wrappings to take blood. He attempts to get a needle into Ben's vein. And then attempts again. Soon Ben's arm is like a pin cushion as the stubborn veins refuse to rise to the surface. Meanwhile his pulse is still registering 29bpm. Something tells me it shouldn't be this low. It's ridiculously low, abnormally low, dangerously low…

A senior doctor arrives, rolls up his sleeves and finally - carefully, oh so carefully - manages to get the needle into Ben's arm. It's a huge needle; such a big needle for such a stick-thin arm. By now the tears are streaming down Ben's thin white face. He looks terrified. He's had some pretty hair-raising things done in his time, what with in-growing toenails, several teeth out and various bone fractures, but this is the first time I've seen him cry in public since he was a small child.

A zillion thoughts rush through my head from *I must ring his dad* to *this is my only child and this is his only heart…* I gaze at him - my beautiful son looking frightened and bewildered, and so very young, these days much younger than his 16 years.

How the heck did my big burly rugby playing son end up here? How did we get from *there* - charging up and down the rugby pitch, Number 3 in the team, a position given to the biggest, toughest boys - to *here* - a gaunt, waif-like Ben lying weak and sick, his heart doing "funny things"? Thin Ben who is starving himself to… Damn it, I refuse to let myself go there.

The crazy thing is that I could save his life. I could get all that lost weight back on in a matter of weeks, maybe even faster. And the even crazier thing is that it should be so ridiculously easy. It seems grotesque - criminal, even - that I am sitting here, in England, in the 21st century, watching my son fade away from malnutrition while bucket-loads of food are all around us. Huge, massive, obscene mountains of food. Cakes, ice cream, bread, pies, puddings, pizzas, curries… Up the road are three enormous supermarkets with shelves piled high with every food imaginable. Down the road are restaurants and take-outs specialising in every cuisine on the planet. Yet my son refuses to eat. Or at least he refuses to eat anything other than the bare minimum needed to keep him alive. I want to punch the wall. I want to kick, scream and shout. I want to get the medical staff to force-feed him and insist that he stuffs his face with life-giving food, even pop a funnel down his throat and pour it all into him. *Why the heck aren't they doing this?* No-one appears terribly concerned about the anorexia…

In fact, right from the start, no-one seems to have treated this as an urgent case. Now, at the end of January 2010, almost four months since I first took Ben to see our GP, we are still waiting for treatment. No-one seems interested. No-one has taken this seriously. And no-one has given us any assistance, advice or support.

I feel as if I'm going to faint. Someone must have noticed because they hand me a glass of water. I'm hot one minute and ice cold the next, still in the surreal bubble that has become our normal world over the last six months or so.

I pull myself together and call my husband Paul who's working about two hours' drive away. "I don't think there's anything to worry about, but…" Paul's on his way. It might be a couple of hours before he gets here, but at least he's on his way.

I make my way back to Ben who appears to be in the process of being moved. I get a fleeting sense of relief. *Is everything okay? Can we go home now?* No, he's being transferred to the other hospital, the one in the city centre - the one with the specialist cardio unit.

Inside my head the dread and panic is unbearable, but I hope it doesn't show. "See you in a bit!" I say with a light-hearted grin as they wheel Ben to the waiting ambulance. I give him a friendly wave, no different (I hope) from the one I'd give if I was dropping him off at the cinema or a friend's house. *Don't want to worry him…*

I dash to the car park, fishing in my bag for my keys, cursing the other hospital for having some of the worst hospital car parking in the country. I decide to call a cab. They can send a car in 90 minutes. Damn it. Eventually I find a cab that can be with me in 20 minutes. It's the longest 20 minutes of my life. Then it takes another 20 minutes to battle through the rush hour traffic. The entire process takes well over an hour but it seems so much longer…

Please let Ben be okay…

2

six months earlier

WE SHOULD HAVE PICKED up on it sooner.

But it isn't until the early autumn of 2009 that the penny finally drops that our only child, Ben, is developing anorexia. When you have a son, especially a sporty, food-loving son, you don't expect them to get anorexia. Not that my husband Paul and I have ever given it any thought. At this point eating disorders are about as far off our radar as you can get.

So, in the July, when 15 year old Ben's passion for exercise and healthy eating starts to go extreme, and he begins to lose weight, we assume it's just a teenage phase. So far we've got off lightly. Despite joking that Ben would turn into a moody monster at the stroke of midnight on his 13th birthday, the "teenage angst" never materialised. Until recently, that is, when he's become a bit more sullen and argumentative - and increasingly obsessed with his appearance.

Sometimes I find him leaning forward and prodding his washboard stomach claiming he's "fat". Or examining his face critically from every angle in the mirror.

I tell him not to be ridiculous. The idea that our son could be sliding into something far more sinister than just "angst" doesn't register. It doesn't register with Ben, either, because it isn't as if he's sat down one day and said, "I'm going to get anorexia". None of us has the slightest idea what is happening and, by the time the penny drops, Ben is already being dragged under fast.

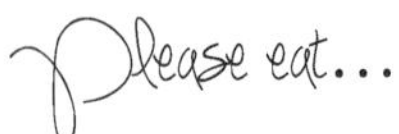

IT'S THE BEGINNING OF JULY, just a couple of weeks before the alarm bells begin to faintly ring in my head. Ben is representing his *house* in the school sports day, running in the 1500 metres against his friend Kieran.

Ben appears confident and self-assured, determined to win. Yet I'm aware that there's still a bit of the inner critic inside his head that always manages to rob him of his new-found confidence - a legacy from primary school. The days when Ben would invariably be the one at the back of the race, plodding along reluctantly, visibly heavier than the other boys. The days when Ben would rather play quietly in a corner of the playground with his friend Peter than kick a ball around the yard. The days before Ben took up sport.

How different Ben looks now. I doubt if his former teachers and school mates would recognise the tall, handsome, athletic young man who's about to win the 1500 metres. The whole of his *house* is cheering as he hurtles past Kieran to the finish line, his arms raised in triumph, reminding me of last summer when he completed the gruelling 140 mile Coast2Coast cycle ride with his dad. I remember the photos we took just before this, in France. Little me standing beside a much taller and broader Ben, my whole being bursting with pride as a group of girls walked past pretending not to glance back at the tanned teenager with the awesome physique and good looks. *Is it my imagination or has he lost a bit of weight since then?*

I make a mental note to make sure he doesn't get any slimmer; it doesn't suit him. Last year the rugby coach moved him from Number 3 ("meat-head and fat", as Ben put it) to Number 8 ("meat-head and not fat") as his body got taller and leaner. They'll have to move him again if he's not careful. But there are two months to go before the rugby season, plenty of time for Ben to bulk out again.

Meanwhile I'm so proud of his victory I could explode. You know who I wish was here now? Timothy, the new boy who joined Ben's primary school in Year 4: lanky, curly haired Timothy who turned Ben's final year at that school into hell.

At first we thought that Timothy was another Peter, Ben's closest friend during the early years of primary school. Both Ben and Peter were quiet, studious and had vivid imaginations. They'd lose themselves in a fantasy world inhabited by exotic creatures. Peter's bed would become a submarine, tank or the gondola of an airship and, on sleepovers, the boys would go late night zombie-hunting around Peter's huge house. As the boys grew older, it was Peter's dad who suggested Ben accompany Peter to Sunday morning mini rugby. Peter gave up after just one session, but - to our surprise - the sports-shy Ben stayed on and quickly became a star player. Then one day Peter moved away and Ben was left on his own.

Not long after this Timothy joined the school. Ben immediately made friends with him. And, as I watched the boys play happily together, I was confident that the gap left by Peter's departure had been filled.

As time went on, however, Paul and I began to notice a distinct change in Ben's frame of mind at weekends. On Sunday evenings his mood plummeted and you could guarantee that he wouldn't sleep that night. He began to drag his feet on Monday mornings and we couldn't figure out why. After all, Ben had always loved school. Then one Sunday it all came to a head when we found him sobbing on the stairs. Ben was being bullied. Snide remarks, whispered insults, unpleasant teasing, pushes and shoves... Timothy was making Ben's life hell.

I remember striding into school and insisting something was done immediately. The Deputy Head promised to have a quiet word with Timothy who, she was certain, had no idea of the effect he was having on Ben, but she'd ask him to apologise anyway. "Then the boys can shake hands and forget about it."

So the boys shook hands. But Timothy didn't forget. He simply went underground. The snide remarks and threats became more secretive. The pushing and shoving were done out of teachers' sight. Nothing changed. If anything it got worse. And the staff still refused to believe that the impeccably behaved Timothy was a bully.

We offered to move Ben to another school. But he insisted on staying put. "I've been here since the start and Timothy's only been here since Year 4. I'm not leaving, not now." I had to hand it to him, Ben had guts.

So now, as Ben flies across the finish line, I wish that Timothy could see him: made-from-concrete, rugby-playing Ben, being cheered on by the whole school. Or, rather, I wish Ben could bump into Timothy and punch his lights out.

My mind rewinds back to those unpleasant days at primary school. By the time Ben sat his 11-plus exam in the January of Year 6 (and won an academic scholarship to a fabulous independent secondary school) the bullying had sapped him of every ounce of confidence and self-esteem. Our GP referred Ben for counselling. It didn't work. The counsellor seemed more interested in my background, implying that I'd passed on my anxieties and insecurities to Ben. No wonder, she implied, Ben had allowed himself to be bullied. These counselling sessions, she said, would be used to toughen Ben up to face the bigger, more daunting world of senior school which, she implied, could be a serious shock to the system for the ill-equipped.

But far from being a shock to the system, Ben took to secondary school like a duck to water. No, it wasn't perfect, but at least Timothy wasn't there. Almost immediately, a super group of boys took Ben under their wing. Ben thrived, and - before long - he'd become one of the most popular boys in his social group. I remember thinking how most parents dread their child getting in with the wrong crowd. Thankfully Ben couldn't have gotten in with a nicer bunch of boys.

Ben's new school had a reputation for sport, especially rugby. It quickly became clear that Ben had a natural talent for the game. He was immediately snapped up for the rugby team and given the position of Number 3, a position given to the biggest, toughest boys. Soon, Ben was playing rugby virtually every day of the week, including local club rugby on Sundays. Before long all the puppy fat disappeared to be replaced with an awesome athletic physique. Over the next four years Ben would transform from the quiet, overweight, bullied boy of primary school into an athletic, confident and popular teenager. We couldn't have wished for more.

Being good at sport carried a distinct kudos and Ben began to revel in the attention he was getting. As "the guy in the rugby team" Ben also had a natural shield against any potential bullying.

"Basically it earned me respect," he'd tell me much later. "For instance if any of the other rugby guys were throwing their weight around in the common room and annoying my friends, I'd tell them to shut up and they would. Instantly. Everyone listened to me."

Back then I remember Ben being involved in a plethora of activities: drama productions, the choir, a band and of course sport. He was also excelling in the classroom, winning various merit awards and a prize on Prize Day. Meanwhile his popularity continued to grow.

Ben's birthday parties were legendary. His birthday is on the 23rd December and so, to avoid having a party right on top of Christmas, a get-together was usually scheduled for the last weekend of term.

Even though Ben's attic bedroom is huge, we had to split the sleepover into two shifts: one set of boys on the Friday night and another on the Saturday. That's how popular Ben was.

The first group would disappear up to Ben's room, only coming down for supplies of drinks, potato crisps, biscuits and cakes and, of course, an enormous evening meal followed by the world's biggest breakfast. After all, they were growing teenage boys, weren't they?

Saturday afternoon was the switch-over when we'd meet up with the other group at the cinema, watch a movie and go to a pizza restaurant (the kind where you help yourself to endless ice cream and sprinkles which, of course, they all did). Then the whole sleepover process would begin again followed by more supplies of biscuits, drinks and potato crisps plus an equally enormous breakfast on Sunday morning. No wonder they say teenage boys have hollow legs.

BEN'S 15TH BIRTHDAY PARTY in December 2008 is the liveliest of all. By this time Ben is at the peak of his popularity and confidence. There's so much noise, bumping, crashing and thumping going on in our attic that I'm worried it will bring the house down. The boys are constantly eating as usual. Well, what do you expect? They're teenage boys after all… I dig out yet another family size bag of potato crisps and some packets of cookies for Ben to take up the two flights of stairs to his room.

After Christmas I'm vaguely aware that Ben has put on a few pounds. Not unusual, I figure, considering how much we've eaten over the festive season. But I know that, once back on the sports field, Ben's weight will level out again - and it does. What I don't know is that, for quite some time now, the green shoots of something sinister have been sprouting in Ben's head. Deep down in the inner recesses of his mind, Ben is busy weighing up input and output in a bid to maintain the athletic physique he's acquired in recent years.

Acutely aware that he's put on weight over Christmas, the next six months will be a constant struggle to stay slim. Extra pounds, Ben's convinced, could easily transport him back to the overweight, bullied boy of primary school. Yet he feels driven to binge. Unbeknown to us he'll devour entire packets of biscuits or chocolates in one sitting and then make himself do a lengthy run to burn it off, returning exhausted. Exercise, he believes, is what is keeping the dreaded pounds at bay. But, increasingly, Ben is feeling lazy. He's had enough of all this sport and he's getting weary of rugby. And I can tell. One

Saturday we drive up to Durham to watch his team play against the local school. Ben's lost his enthusiasm. He slouches around, complaining of a tummy ache and eventually gets invalided off the pitch. I can sense the coach getting irritated.

Meanwhile Ben is convinced there must be a better, easier way to stay slim rather than thrashing it out on a freezing cold, muddy rugby pitch every day of the week. He's already secretly experimenting with food. But Paul and I scarcely notice what's going on. We put the growing fussiness down to "being a teenager". Ben didn't develop an attitude at 13 but, by golly, he seems to be heading that way now…

But on that sports day afternoon in July 2009 Ben is in a euphoric mood. As Paul and I watch him streak across the finish line, all we see is a boy who's thriving in every way. Good grief, at one point last term I even toyed with the idea of writing to the Headmaster to congratulate him on how the school had been the making of Ben.

In the event I will end up contacting the Headmaster about something altogether different… something I could never in a million years imagine we would have a conversation about.

3

health kick

IT'S LATE JULY, A WEEK OR so after Ben's victory at sports day. We're in France, relaxing around the pool of the villa we've rented near Cognac. Ben is swimming up and down. Up, down, up, down… until he's counted to one hundred. He does this every day; he's a keen swimmer. Or at least that's how it still looks to us. After all, he did the same last summer and the summer before. He's also jogging through the vines to the little crossroads and back every morning. He didn't do that last year. There's a ripple of anxiety somewhere deep inside my mind, but little more than that.

Ben is also on a healthy eating kick - something which I'm vaguely aware began in the spring.

"Give it a break, Ben," I say as he refuses another ice cream. "We're on holiday. Everyone has ice creams on holiday!" I've also noticed that he isn't eating the crisps we always bring on our picnics. "Have a biscuit," I offer, "Or a banana?" "No I'm fine," he replies. This concerns me because I'm aware that he hasn't had very much breakfast: some bread and jam (no butter) and black coffee. *When, I wonder, did he start drinking black coffee?*

Ben's never been fussy about food. Not up to now, at any rate. When he was a baby he drank milk as if it was going out of fashion. As a child he revelled in the home-cooked meals I'd make him: nutritionally packed burgers with "spooky mash", cheesy semolina fingers, vegetable sausages and all manner of other creative meals, always followed by a pudding. If Ben's tea - which he'd have earlier than Paul and me - wasn't ready on time he'd get quite agitated and, for some time, I remember feeling anxious if his food wasn't on the table by 5 o'clock.

Ben loved school dinners and usually went back for second helpings. He would have had thirds, too, if he could. He also loved to eat out, especially in country pubs where he would hoover up whatever child's meal was on the menu. I used to look at the meagre child's portion of fish fingers and chips, or whatever, and know it wouldn't satisfy Ben's man-sized appetite. So I wasn't surprised when he graduated to adult portions far sooner than most children. I'd watch with admiration as he'd demolish every single morsel. No fussiness, no pushing the food around the plate like other kids. He'd eat most of my leftovers, too, and an adult-sized pudding.

Dinners at secondary school weren't quite as exciting as primary school, but that didn't stop Ben from tucking in. Then, one summer, the canteen was given a complete revamp and a professional chef brought in to makeover the menu. Gone were the pies, chips and beans to be replaced by gourmet menus and a healthy new salad bar. The food was out of this world. I expected foodie Ben to be in culinary heaven.

But increasingly over the past six months, Ben has been opting for the salad bar. Or a bowl of soup and a roll, followed by fruit. Or - unbeknown to me - even less if he's going to be "sitting down doing nothing all afternoon". I'm convinced he's missing out on the best school dinners in the country. "But, mum," he's always reminding me, "I come home to a huge evening meal every night. Most of my friends just grab a sandwich in front of the telly". Nowadays the three of us eat a home-cooked meal in the dining room every evening.

In a way having a smaller lunch makes sense to me. Personally I'm not too keen on eating a huge meal at lunchtime and feeling sleepy all afternoon. But I have no idea that Ben is cutting back on breakfast, too. Sometimes he'll just have a quick slice of toast or a banana. Some days he doesn't have anything at all. So he's eating minimally until our evening meal while continuing to do the usual sporting activities. But I don't see this. Not until our French holiday when his tweaked eating becomes more noticeable because we're with him all the time.

As Paul watches Ben complete another run past the vineyards he offers to buy him gym membership when we get home - the perfect preparation for the new rugby season in September. Ben thinks it's a great idea and begins to flick through the men's health and fitness magazines he's brought with him.

On the way back to the ferry port we stop off for a night in the Loire Valley. There's a photo of Ben and me standing on the balcony of a chateau: Ben with his mirrored aviator sunglasses hooked into the top of his tee-shirt, leather thong necklace, hair carefully puttied into spikes, hands in the pockets of his khaki shorts. Ben looks cool. But I'm sure he looks a little leaner than he did this time last year. I put it down to natural body changes.

BACK IN ENGLAND Ben embraces the gym with enthusiasm, especially the cardio machines. Every day he jogs up to the gym and back, his face flushed, pleased with himself at his staying power. He's also doing lengthy runs and can be out for an hour at a time. Then he'll flick through the men's health magazines until he comes to the diets and exercises that promise to deliver bodies like the defined muscle men featured in the pages.

I'm not sure I feel too comfortable about Ben reading these magazines. I'm convinced they're making him over-critical as he compares himself to the impossibly toned models.

"You look amazing," I reassure him as he examines his abs, arms, thighs and rear in the mirror. "I beg to differ," he responds, looking back at his reflection critically.

One evening he's sitting on the sofa with his eyes on his belly rather than the TV. I can tell he's preoccupied. It's something that's happening more and more. He pulls up his tee-shirt and bends forward so the skin on his belly falls into natural folds. He pinches it between his thumb and forefinger, and then tries to grab it with his fist. "Rolls of fat," he says, dully, grabbing more skin.

"Ben, that's just skin," I point out. "Everyone's stomach does that, even the men in those magazines." But, for some reason, he can't see it and it bothers me. "And what does it matter?" I add for good measure.

To deflect his attention from the body checking I suggest he invites his friends round, reminding him that he hasn't seen them since school broke up for the summer vacation.

"What the hell would we do?" he asks blankly.

"Meet in town, go to the cinema, a meal or whatever… the usual stuff?"

His eyes are fixed his belly. "They're always busy and, anyway, they're boring - and most of them are on holiday." This summer he seems to prefer the gym to his friends and it concerns me. Not for the first time do I wish Ben's friends lived locally rather than miles away. Get-togethers need to be arranged via mobiles or Facebook.

But recently I haven't noticed Ben rushing to do either.

4

chopping fruit

IT'S AUGUST AND BEN IS BUSY in the kitchen. Last night we had wine, oil and thyme roasted butternut squash stuffed with Moroccan couscous plus a watercress and tomato salad with horseradish dressing. On Saturday it was melt-in-the-mouth griddled rump steaks with a fiery pepper sauce and mushroom and pimiento side, accompanied by fresh aromatic herb and olive oil bread. There's even a breakfast option of blueberry and apricot muffins with chopped fresh fruit and yoghurt. In fact the only thing that hasn't been a massive success is the evil-smelling sourdough bread that I wouldn't wish on my worst enemy.

Meanwhile cookery books are the new computer games as Ben makes long lists of what he's going to cook next. "You won't need to cook for the next 12 months, mum!" he tells me indulgently.

"Suits me," I say, brain-dead from umpteen years of slaving over a hot stove. I'm a pretty good cook. But, to be truthful, he's better than me.

Ben loves to watch TV cookery programmes. Tonight it's *River Cottage*. We've already watched the *Hairy Bikers* and *Jamie Oliver*, and we never miss *Nigella* or *Nigel Slater*. Then there are all those programmes about what you should and shouldn't eat to stay healthy. Ben particularly loves the ones where they take an obese person and examine a typical week's food intake. The horrified look on Ben's face is a picture as they pour chips, crisps, cakes, cola, sweets, chocolates, cookies, pizzas and a mountain of other "baddies" into a perspex tube. Or they spread it out on a table for everyone to see and gasp in horror. This kind of programme makes us both feel incredibly smug and self-righteous with our healthy home-cooked meals.

Ben has even started to love aubergines, courgettes and mushrooms, the only foods he never really liked. I am now in the enviable position of having a teenager that will eat anything. Well *almost* anything. He's not keen on things with too much fat or calories in them. Sometimes I wish they'd ban those darn nutritional labels because Ben seems more interested in them than in the food the packaging contains. *When on earth did Ben become interested in calories?* Good God, the word "calorie" shouldn't even feature in a teenage boy's vocabulary.

The more I think about it the more I feel as if Ben's become a kind of "food policeman". If I want to treat myself to goodies like biscuits or chocolate I have to literally sneak them into the house and hide them. If he catches me… well… boy, am I in trouble! When he comes shopping with me he whips the offending items out of the trolley and back onto the shelf - choc-chip soft-bake cookies being the latest casualty that never made it to my mouth. ("You don't need those, mum!" he barks. "Yes I do," I plead. "I've had a bad day…") I'm vaguely irritated. After all, I'm supposed to be the boss, not him.

He's already planning what we're going to eat at Christmas: sushi plus healthy things in filo pastry. Oh and he's even offering to cook Christmas dinner. But no mince pies, chocolate logs, gooey creamy goodies or Christmas cake as we could all do with going on a health kick. So Ben says.

Meanwhile whatever I need from the cupboard or fridge has vanished, absorbed into the latest culinary delight. Talk about teenage boys eating you out of house and home…

The trouble is… I don't think Ben *is* eating us out of house and home; it's Paul and me who are doing most of the eating. Ben is just doing the cooking. But he always seems to be there, armed with another tray of something mouth-watering, insisting we sample it while he looks on like an indulgent grandma. "Try this, mum!" he'll say pushing a spoonful of whatever it is towards my face, refusing to take no for an answer. "Go on, go on!" The laden spoon gets so close I can't focus my eyes on it. I have no option but to open my mouth and taste.

Sometimes I feel so full I can't eat another bite. I especially love the potato focaccia he's just baked. It's fantastic with butter. Any worries I may have about Ben cutting back on food are promptly put on a back burner as he shovels this into his mouth, slice after luscious slice. But what I don't know is that, inside his head, something is already beating him up for getting out of control and "pigging out". It's a voice that is about to get louder. Much louder.

When Ben's not cooking, he's busy re-writing our cookery books. He looks almost saintly in his white apron as he conjures up yet another calorie and fat stripped meal or bake. ("See? You *can* make cakes without fat!"... "Why fry onions in oil when you can dry fry? It's so much healthier, mum.")

I'm reminded of the slimming magazine I used to buy in the 1970s with its Thin Twin recipes: re-worked with clever little calorie saving tricks like replacing half the meat with grated carrot, lightly spraying the pan with oil rather than slugging it in, using corn starch to make a cheese sauce rather than the traditional butter and flour (with half fat cheese naturally...)

"Look!" he exclaims with enthusiasm as we go round the local supermarket. "They're doing an 'extra light' mayonnaise now!" Ping - into our trolley it goes, having passed the fat and calorie content test with flying colours. Sometimes it seems as if he's hijacked the entire supermarket shopping experience. And the kitchen, too. He's making the shopping lists, organising the menus, even re-arranging the fridge and cupboard contents. ("Don't you mess it up, mum, or I'll be furious!") He's begun to watch me when I'm eating. Like a hawk. If I leave anything on my plate he comes down on me like a ton of bricks and I'm sick of repeating, "I'm a middle-aged woman, I'm only 5ft 3, I don't need to eat as much as a growing teenage boy!"

"Don't eat that, you'll spoil your evening meal!" Ben snaps as I reach for the biscuit jar. Yet again I feel irritation, but this time it's tinged with something else that I can't put my finger on.

Meanwhile the running has become more rigorous and the gym visits more frequent, supplemented by sit-ups, press-ups and crunches, plus a daily yoga session. I'm impressed with his dedication. But something at the back of my mind clicks in with *This isn't normal...*

Is it my imagination or is Ben losing weight? So I say: "You realise that all this extra exercise means you should be eating much more than you are?" But he just shrugs it off, reminding me of how easily he puts on weight and insisting that he, with his body makeup and "low metabolism", doesn't need "loads of" food. And anyway he's still a teenager, not a grown man.

"I don't want to get fat," he says, "You know what I was like as a kid".

Or the more hurtful "Mum, why did you feed me so much when I was a kid?" to which I immediately snap: "I didn't; you loved your food and made my life hell if you didn't get it!"

Then I add: "With all this exercise and healthy eating there's as much chance of you getting fat as there is of me winning the lottery." I remind him that lots of young children have puppy fat. "And, anyway, you're different now. Your body has changed." I tell him I'm worried he isn't eating properly and is losing weight.

Ben looks at me aghast, as if I've just made the most ridiculous comment in the universe. "Mum, I've got a gut! And a double chin! Look!" He prods the offending areas. All I see is skin.

Alright, I think, I'll prove to him how much he needs to eat with all this exercise. I send off for a book - a "bible" of sports nutrition - and point out the calorie-laden eating plans on its pages. "If you're doing weights, running, rowing and bikes you need to be eating at least *this much* every day." I point to page after page of charts. But Ben scarcely looks at them. He knows better.

All he seems bothered about is the damage that high levels of saturated fat can do to his body. It has become Public Enemy Number One. He refuses to eat anything with even a hint of saturated fat in it. And, before long, all the other fats have been thrown into the baddies basket, too. Fat is bad. Fat must be avoided at all costs. I'm painfully aware that Ben's whittling down the list of foods he will eat to the bare minimum: fruit, vegetables, salad and diet foods.

FAST-FORWARD TO THE present day. I'm beginning to put this book together and am talking to Ben about these crucial months between his 15th birthday and the end of summer 2009.

What prompts this is a photo of Ben and his friends taken at that birthday party. There's stuff everywhere; bedding, snacks, games consoles, all the usual things you'd expect in a boy's bedroom. A flushed Ben is standing on the left, smiling, hands in pockets - just a normal boy messing around with his mates. Earlier on, I remember, they'd been spraying each other with the shower hose and making a terrible racket.

"Inside I was feeling fat, flabby and greedy," he tells me. "I'd just eaten an entire box of chocolates in one sitting. Given half the chance I'd eat anything in one go and then make myself do a 60-minute run to wear it off, come back exhausted and have to sit down all afternoon because I was knackered."

He tells me how he began to get depressed, "constantly swinging from a real high to a real low; from eating loads to eating next to nothing. It wasn't a new thing, though; I'd been like this for years - all or nothing. I found it hard to work out a middle ground. Food made me feel happy. But I began to feel I needed to 'earn' it otherwise I wasn't 'allowed' it. And I started skipping breakfasts, but then I'd mess it all up by having huge puddings in the evening and stuff, which is why - at that early stage - I wasn't losing weight, so you didn't notice anything. I had no idea what was happening to me. I was so mixed up, but I thought it was just part of being a teenager".

When Ben first took up rugby, he enjoyed it. "It was fun, but as time went on it became like a millstone around my neck. I was fed up with it, but too scared to stop in case I put on weight. All that hard work for nothing; I couldn't face that. Then I began to look at the nutritional content of food and was horrified at the amount of calories I was eating. Heck, back then I didn't even know that whipped cream contained fat - I thought it was whipped milk! So I had a bit of a think. First I'd cut back on stuff like breakfasts and school dinners. Then I figured that, by switching to low fat or no fat options, I could eat the same quantity but do less exercise. What you were seeing over that summer, mum, was me re-writing recipes and producing fat-free bakes so I could stuff my face without getting fat."

"So," I say, "it felt like the proverbial 'magic bullet'?"

"Yep, but the irony was that instead of exercising less I began to exercise more than ever: press-ups, sit-ups, you name it. And it continued to shock me how many calories were in things; stuff I used to eat without a second thought. Ice cream, biscuits, crisps… I began a mental black list of foods I wouldn't eat. Also, one of the reasons I'd stopped seeing my friends over that summer was because I knew they'd often end up in a burger or pizza bar, and that kind of place was a total no-go area for me."

ONE AFTERNOON BEN ARRIVES back from the gym in a foul mood. I'm getting used to opening the front door and bracing myself for the latest tale of woe.

"Talk to me, Ben," I insist as he walks wordlessly past me like a zombie. "Tell me what's wrong - maybe I can help."

He rests his head against the hallway mirror, fists against the wall. Gradually he begins to emit a long, low roar, like an animal in pain, flicking his head round to stare me in the face. I haven't seen him like this before.

"Mum, can't you see?" he shrieks, flailing his arms around like he used to do as a toddler. "I hate the gym. I hate all this exercise. I hate it, hate it, hate it!" He's beginning to get worked up, almost hysterical.

I'm taken aback. All I can say is "Then why do it? Stop right now. Just stop doing it!"

"I can't, mum! Don't you see? I *can't* stop! I *have* to do it!" Tears are streaming down his reddened face. I can't tell if the penetrating look he's giving me is a cry for help or just hopelessness.

"Right, I'm going to cancel the gym membership," I say as if this will solve the problem. "And I want you to stop all that running. Go out with your friends instead. Have fun!"

But I have a feeling I'm banging my head against a brick wall. Could Ben be addicted to exercise? Like someone can get addicted to drugs or alcohol?

CHOP, CHOP, CHOP. Ben's in the kitchen with bags of assorted dried and fresh fruit. These days we buy an awful lot of fruit. He's been in the kitchen for quite some time, carefully chopping the fruit before arranging it on a small plate. This is his dessert. The next dessert will look identical.

Ben won't let me go to the supermarket alone; making the excuse that he needs to choose his own fruit. But I'm aware that he's scrutinising what I buy more than ever. Everything that goes into the trolley is analysed to make sure it passes the fat and calories test, and if it doesn't, then it goes back onto the shelf. It takes far longer to do the supermarket shopping than it used to. It's also becoming incredibly stressful.

On the occasions when I do manage to sneak to the supermarket alone, I find I'm policing my own shopping. I'd better not buy this or that, because Ben will refuse to eat it. Things like cheese, puff pastry, ice cream, cookies and cake, even semi-skimmed milk are no-no's. Even bread has fat in it, says Ben, so he doesn't eat very much of that either. Better to buy low fat or no fat groceries because at least I know he'll eat them. I'd rather he eat these than nothing at all.

I also find myself flicking through food magazines, discounting the vast majority of recipes. I can't choose that one; it's got cheese in it. Some kind of sauce? Only if it's tomato sauce, and onions must now be dry-fried. Meat? Only if it is one hundred per cent lean. Pastry? Not a chance. Cream? Who are you kidding? Greek yoghurt maybe? Only if it's zero fat. Won't two per cent fat be okay? One per cent, maybe? Unfortunately not.

What's happened to the Ben who would eat anything? The boy who would clean his own plate and proceed to clean ours too?

In fact, watching him chopping up fruit, I've a sneaking suspicion that he's probably eating even less than we think. And I don't understand why, especially as he's doing all this exercise.

"Don't you think Ben's lost a lot of weight?" my mother-in-law remarks when she visits in September. She hasn't seen him since Christmas and I can see by her face she's shocked at the change. "Don't you think he should see a GP?"

That night we eat out at a local country pub. My mother-in-law is watching Ben like a hawk, noting what he does and doesn't eat, and how he's careful about what he chooses from the menu. He's taking awfully long to choose, too, switching from one choice to another, then back again. He's also silent and subdued.

These days he's like this much of the time.

Once she's gone I can't get her words out of my head - or the shocked expression on her face. Suddenly I'm looking at Ben with different eyes. Yes we were aware he was losing weight because of the "healthy eating" and exercise. But I think we were also assuming he'd snap out of it once he was back at school, eating school dinners and playing rugby.

A day or so later, Ben and I spend a day in Liverpool. I'm so relieved to see he's back to his normal, light-hearted self. I'm even more relieved when we order a couple of huge takeout subs from Subway and sit on a bench eating, chatting away, just like old times. We visit the art gallery and I have a coffee in the café afterwards. Ben has a fizzy drink, a non-diet drink I notice. Then at the station we buy the latest Good Food magazine which we read together on the journey home.

It's this kind of event that confuses me, that makes me wonder if I'm worrying over nothing. Is Ben developing a problem? Or is it just a passing teenage phase? Will he bulk out again once he gets back to school dinners and the rugby pitch? I know my mother-in-law suggested we visit the GP. But how can I claim that Ben isn't eating when he clearly is? Or at least he is some of the time. I don't know what to do. I can't decide if there's anything wrong or not.

However Ben is still exercising, despite claiming that he hates it. He's exercising more than ever. And he's still revamping recipes and avoiding certain foods, and policing the kitchen and supermarket shopping. He is also getting thinner. So it wouldn't do any harm to have a chat with the GP. Just to be on the safe side. I make an appointment. The GP can't see us for another week or so.

5

back to school

THE NEW SCHOOL YEAR begins as usual. It's Year 11 - GCSE year - the final year before the sixth form. Ben seems much more subdued than last year. If I thought the hair preening and body checking were bad in the spring, things are 10 times worse now. He seems to be having a bad image day almost every day.

He's spending ages getting ready for school. Everything about his uniform is wrong: blazer too big, sweater too shapeless, shirt too unflattering - and almost immediately we have to buy new trousers as the old ones are far too big. We've been shopping and Ben has bought a girls' school sweater, tight and shaped at the waist, making him look even thinner. Boys' sweaters are too baggy. They make him look "fat", he says.

Every morning I catch him examining himself critically in the full-length mirror, carefully arranging his sweater, shirt and tie, and adjusting his hair which he's already straightened with tongs and messed up with goo.

Please let him be happy with the result, I whisper to myself knowing that if one hair's out of place Ben's mood will flip and he'll take it out on me. Why the heck did I ever suggest buying a bigger blazer so he could "grow into it" rather than one that fitted? He's swamped in it now and, of course, he's blaming me.

Part of me says this is normal 15 year old behaviour. Show me a teenager that isn't rude to their parents, doesn't check their hair and clothes one hundred times in the mirror and doesn't hate wearing school uniform.

But the other part of me says this isn't normal. What's happened to the boy whose birthday parties had to be held in shifts because he was so popular? The boy that sang in a band, watched movies and had fun?

Ben is still not mixing with his friends. "Mum, I feel so disconnected," he says. "I just can't relate to them anymore. And they're always annoying me."

This conversation is repeated almost every evening, like a stuck record. Someone always seems to have wound him up in some way and Ben always seems to be on a downer.

He's even less enthusiastic about rugby. It's the first match of the season and the parents are gathered around the pitch hugging Styrofoam cups of coffee. Some of the boys, including Ben's friend Kieran, have been picked to play for the second team with the sixth form boys. Ben has been picked, too, but I'm worried he doesn't have enough bulk. Not to play alongside 18 year olds built like brick outhouses. What is the coach thinking of? Ben's not keen, either, and tries to get the coach to move him back to the less aggressive third team. The coach has high hopes for Ben and isn't pleased. Something in me wishes the coach would refuse to let him play altogether. Can't he see Ben is too thin for rugby?

This season Ben just doesn't seem to have the stamina he had in the days when he would drive down the pitch like a steam roller, flattening the opposition in his path before hurtling himself and the ball over the touch line to loud cheers. I can't help thinking that if someone tackled him roughly now, he'd snap like a twig. So when he breaks his nose a week or so later and is invalided out of the team it's not a great surprise. In fact it's quite a relief…

AT THE END OF SEPTEMBER I fall sick. Suddenly and without

warning I lose my balance. I feel nauseous and dizzy, as if I'm walking on a ship in high seas. My brain feels like mush. I can't think straight and I certainly can't work. Before long, supermarket shopping becomes a nightmare, too, as the shelves and aisles swim before my eyes. Ben takes over all the cooking and I spend the greater part of each day in bed.

So, in the event, it's me that visits the GP first. But the GP can't find anything wrong. I feel like a fake.

A day or so later I'm back in his surgery, this time with Ben.

"Ben's lost an awful lot of weight recently," I explain. "And he's been doing a lot of exercise over the summer."

The GP looks across at Ben. "Your mum seems to think you're not eating enough. What do *you* think?"

Ben shakes his head and sighs as if humouring me, then smiles and says calmly: "I'm fine. I really don't know what my mum's worrying about." The GP looks over at me, eyebrows raised for my response. I could be imagining it, but I suspect there is a hint of the "over-protective, fussy mother" in that look. Yet again I feel like a fraud.

"Okay, Ben, let's see how much you weigh - and I'll measure your height, too." The GP walks over to the scales and asks Ben to remove his shoes. Ben's weight is low, but not overly so. Not enough to start the alarm bells ringing if you hadn't known him as a big burly rugby player. The GP turns to me for my response. I can't read his expression.

A wave of self-doubt sweeps over me. Does he think I'm making it up? After all, he couldn't find anything wrong with me the other day. And now here I am with my son who doesn't appear to have anything wrong with him either. We're sent away with instructions to "eat sensibly and come back in a couple of weeks". I meekly take Ben home.

A few days later, Ben falls sick with flu-like symptoms and lies in bed groaning with sudden bouts of sobbing. I call the surgery and talk to the nurse.

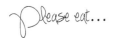

"He's not eating, he's lethargic and he's aching all over," I explain, telling her that he doesn't seem to have a temperature. Could it be flu? The nurse thinks it's probably a virus, but she's not sure, so I take him into the surgery to get checked over. No fever or vomiting, she writes in his notes, but he's lost his appetite and is losing weight.

I've been busy Googling Ben's symptoms. "Do you think he could be developing an eating disorder?" I ask, hoping and praying she'll put my mind at rest. She doesn't appear to be unduly concerned. Am I fussing over nothing? Is it just one of these mysterious 24-hour bugs that disappear as quickly as they came?

Back home Ben's moods are beginning to swing quite violently. One minute he's completely normal and the next he's sobbing uncontrollably, claiming to be freezing cold, then hot, and aching all over. Cramps in his stomach make it uncomfortable to eat. I notice the skin on his hands, especially between the fingers, is dry, scaly and red. I take one of his hands to have a closer look. It's ice cold.

I make two more appointments with the GP: one for Ben and another for me, because my nausea and dizziness are getting worse. The GP notes that Ben feels generally unwell, but - like the nurse - he doesn't think it's a viral infection. I point out that Ben's still not eating properly. We've had to borrow my dad's leather punch to add extra notches to his belt and buy new school trousers. Again I ask if Ben could be developing an eating disorder. The GP makes Ben promise to eat more and we're dispatched off home with some creams for his dry skin. "It's all in your mind!" a voice shouts inside my head.

"I'm here again!" I say, feeling like a fraud as I walk into the GP's surgery the next day. But I manage to get him to refer me to a specialist (who eventually diagnoses a problem with my inner ear).

Then, the following week, it's Ben's turn. This time I book him in with a different GP; I really can't face the other one again.

But Ben's weight has gone up. Damn, part of me says as Ben gives me one of his accusing *See, I said you're being silly* looks. That's put a spanner in the works. I feel as if I'm making a fuss over nothing.

"His mood is getting worse - and so is his behaviour," I tell the GP, hoping this will trigger alarm bells. The GP nods, turns to look at Ben and gives him a short pep talk about sensible eating.

"Starving yourself can seriously damage your body - the parts you can't see, the internal organs and so on," she tells Ben, explaining that he mustn't cut back on food. "At your age you need to put on muscle which means you need to eat sensibly." Then she adds: "If you'd like to see me on your own - without your mum - and just talk about things, then I'll be more than happy to do that. How about in three or four weeks' time? Once you've had time to think through what I've been saying?"

I can sense Ben getting agitated. Suddenly and without warning he stands up and shouts: "I'm fine, there's nothing wrong with me!" He glares at me. "You're just paranoid. I don't know what I'm f*cking doing here" and storms out of the surgery. I get "that look" again from the GP.

I feel helpless. Ben is losing weight fast and behaving strangely. Normally he'd listen to the GP's advice. That's the sort of person Ben is. Or the sort of person he used to be, with impeccable manners and respect for authority. But now he's in complete denial that there's anything wrong. I can't get my head round it. What happens if he continues to lose weight? More and more I'm worrying that, if left unchecked, whatever it is could develop into something serious like anorexia. I mean, anorexia has to begin somewhere, doesn't it? People don't just become skeletal overnight; they have to start losing weight first. Is this how anorexia begins? Is it possible to have anorexia, or at least to be developing anorexia, yet not appear to look much different from anyone else? But, surely, boys don't get anorexia? Or at least I've never heard of a boy getting anorexia. Yet my gut instinct tells me this could be where Ben's heading if someone doesn't take action soon. My blood freezes at the idea.

But Paul and I seem to be the only people that are worried. The GPs don't appear to be. Ben isn't worried, either. He can't see anything wrong. He doesn't seem to realise how drastically his behaviour, mood and physical appearance have changed over the past few months. This isn't like a normal illness or problem where recognisable symptoms are there for all to see: a broken bone, a worrying lump, blood loss or whatever - the sort of issues that GPs deal with on a daily basis. Here I am with a child who - if you hadn't seen him as a stocky rugby player - looks relatively normal, if rather thin. Apart from that there are no visible symptoms. I mean, he doesn't look like a "text book" anorexic. He's not skin and bone; he just looks skinny. Worse, he insists there is nothing wrong with him.

How on earth can I expect the medical profession to take me seriously when even the patient insists they're okay and alleges their mother is imagining it all? Especially when that mother appears to have a curious, unidentifiable illness of her own.

Am I imagining it? Is it all in my mind? Am I going crazy? I am seriously beginning to wonder…

6

six pack

OVER THE NEXT FEW WEEKS our family life undergoes a complete shift from being a normal family to being a family coping with a nightmare. Unless you've been through it, you won't believe how quickly an eating disorder can creep up on a person. The emerging realisation that your healthy, happy teenage child is developing anorexia is like a horror story unfolding before your eyes. And, by the time you realise something is very seriously wrong, they're already ensnared. By mid-October 2009 Ben has transformed into someone we don't recognise. One day it suddenly dawns on me that I am terrified of my own child.

Anorexia has taken over Ben. Anorexia has taken over our family. And anorexia isn't just about eating; it's about a host of other things - like depression, panic, zero self-esteem and much, much more. I don't just mean feeling a "bit low" now and again; I mean deep, dark depression and self-hatred. I mean banging your head against a wall or thumping your fists against your skull, throwing things around and animal howling… that sort of depression.

With anorexia it's as if someone else takes over your mind. Someone that taunts you all the time, telling you you're fat and that you'll never be popular until you get thin.

Anorexia has you pinching the skin on your skinny stomach, taunting you that it's rolls of flab. Anorexia makes you exercise like crazy and examine yourself over-critically in the mirror. Anorexia makes you hate what you see. Anorexia lies to you that it can make you ultra-handsome, ultra-popular and ultra-confident. If you get thin. It's the ultimate carrot dangling in front of your eyes.

Anorexia lies that it can put you in control of your life. And part of this control is to control exactly what goes into your stomach, how much of it and when. The minute you deviate from this rigid eating pattern, anorexia lies to you that you're out of control. Just one serving of dinner that's not the "right size" and anorexia can have the sufferer banging their head on the fridge and screaming. I know, because this is what Ben is doing virtually every day by late autumn 2009.

With anorexia, it's as if your child becomes two distinctly different beings: their normal self - the child you've known, nurtured and loved since birth - and "the anorexia" - a terrifying, domineering bully that torments both child and parent. An alternate personality that's hell-bent on destruction, a "thing" that transforms your child's behaviour, mannerisms, facial expressions, even voice tone and pitch. Often in an instant. Like flicking a switch. And, the deeper Ben gets sucked into this illness, the more frequently this alternate personality kicks in.

Many people with anorexia give this "thing" a name. The anorexia is often referred to as AN (Anorexia Nervosa) or ED (Eating Disorder). One parent I read about describes anorexia as like having a goblin perched on his daughter's shoulder. Some people even think of anorexia as a kind of "demon". Yes, I decide, that's what it's like. A demon.

The Anorexia Demon.

Looking at family photographs is a painful, instant reminder of what Ben used to look like and should look like, but no longer does. We used to have a big, burly rugby player for a son. Now we have a ghostly waif whose mood is becoming so volatile I am terrified of what he will do next.

One morning I'm standing in the hallway waiting to take Ben to the school bus. "Ben!" I shout up the stairwell for the umpteenth time. "We're going to miss it!"

My muscles tense the moment I've said those words. It's a physical reaction I will become familiar with over the next few months. I feel like a tightly coiled spring.

Almost every morning I'll hear a sudden crash as something is thumped or kicked upstairs, or a door is slammed shut. Often there's a guttural growling that rises in volume to be rounded off with a string of shrieked obscenities. If Ben makes it downstairs he'll continue swearing and shouting, or he'll break down sobbing - Ben who never used to swear in his life.

Sometimes he'll yell and crash around so much that I feel like slapping him across the face like they used to do to hysterical women in the old black-and-white movies. Instead, I just scream and scream at him to calm down. If, that is, I can make my voice louder than his. I slam the front door closed. It's only 7.15 in the morning and our street is eerily silent. I suspect they can hear us on the other side of town. They can certainly hear us next door. After all, we live in a semi-detached house and share a party wall. I can hear them tinkling on the piano or pushing the vacuum cleaner around. God only knows what they're thinking now… They probably think I'm killing him. By the time I eventually get Ben into the car his distress is agonising. And we're not even at the school bus stop yet, let alone school…

Some days I get the silent treatment where he sits in the passenger seat, staring straight ahead as if in some kind of terrible trance. To be truthful, I'm not sure which is worse, that or the screaming and violence. At the bus stop he slams the car door so viciously I'm frightened it will fall off. I feel as if I'm being punished, but I'm not sure what for. Why is he taking it out on me? But taking *what* out on me? That's what I don't understand. What is wrong with Ben? Okay every parent experiences a bit of hassle getting their children ready for school in the morning, but this is a completely different kettle of fish.

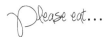

Ben slouches off down the hill to the bus stop where he stands apart from the other kids. Sometimes he runs down the hill still in tears. And all the time I'm coiled up like a spring, primed for the next onslaught.

I dread him coming home. I used to look forward to picking him up from school and listening to all the news and gossip. Now he seems to be in a permanently unpleasant mood, returning with tales of how so-and-so annoyed him or everyone's been ignoring him. I say the obvious: "Well what do you expect if you ignored your friends all summer?" No response. I'm beginning to get used to Ben storming up to his bedroom and slamming the door, followed by a crash of some sort as he thumps something.

Is it my imagination or is he exercising more than ever? Broken nose or no broken nose, he still seems to be able to fill up the week with some kind of physical activity.

"I'M JUST NOT HUNGRY," he says, pushing the food to the side of his plate at the evening meal. "I had a massive lunch."

I have no idea that he's only eaten a few lettuce leaves and an apple. I also have no idea that he is so ravenous he could eat a horse, but he's forcing himself to have just enough to quell the hunger pangs and then stop. When the pangs start again, as they do very soon, what I will come to recognise as the "anorexia voice" - the "inner critic on steroids" inside his head - tells him not to be so greedy.

"Aren't you starving after all that running?" I ask one evening in the careful way I'm beginning to master these days. Ben has joined the cross country club which runs after school a couple of times a week and which he's embraced with an almost religious fervour. I have no idea where the new, thinner Ben finds the energy. I feel uneasy about him doing it. Why are the coaches allowing it? Can't they see he's too thin?

"Mum, I had a big lunch," he says. And for once it's true. If I'd been a fly on the wall in the school canteen, I would have seen him tucking into a proper hot meal for a change - or devouring a large slice of millionaire's shortbread for dessert.

That, he'll tell me years later, is because he knew he'd be running after school and had "earned the right" to eat.

And meanwhile something inside his head is goading him to run faster and further. Yet, because his body isn't getting enough fuel, it's becoming harder to do. But he has to keep on going because if he stops he'll get fat. Or at least that's what this "thing" inside his head tells him.

With a heavy heart I decide it's time to "come clean" and explain to the school that Ben isn't himself at the moment. I call the Head of Year and warn him that Ben's behaving unusually and may begin to do "strange things". We're not entirely sure what's wrong, but he's lost so much weight recently that we think it may be an eating disorder. We're waiting for a diagnosis.

The teacher isn't surprised; he's already noticed the dramatic weight loss and so have half the PE staff. After all, Ben is involved in just about every sport in the school. They are worried. Seriously worried.

IT'S A GOOD THING I came clean. Very soon I begin to get regular emergency phone calls from school asking me to come and pick up the pieces of whatever chaos the emerging eating disorder has driven Ben to create that day. I begin to dread the school's name showing up on my phone. Usually it's Sheila - the school nurse - that gets in touch.

I'm getting used to dashing around for my car keys, heading off to school and rushing into the reception area. "I'm just off to see Sheila, she's expecting me." I make my way to the medical centre, climbing the stone staircase, past the library and through the fire doors. "Knock, knock," I announce, pushing open the door. Sheila greets me with a hug. "Come in, dear, and sit down," she says, asking if I'd like a coffee.

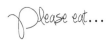

Instantly I feel safe. I glance up at the mantelpiece above the boarded-up fireplace. There's an assortment of trinkets, teddy bears and thank you cards. Behind me is a squishy sofa and through the archway are four iron bedsteads made up for emergencies. Through the tall sash windows with their old hand-made glass I can see the rose garden and cricket pitch, and beyond that the rugby fields and the woods rising up from the river. The glass makes the trees look wiggly and for a moment I'm distracted...

Sheila's voice nudges me back to reality. Ben is missing some of his lessons, she says. "The thing is... if the register says he's in school we need to know where he is." Usually Ben can be found hiding in the boys' toilets and Sheila will calm him down in the medical centre. These days it takes an awful lot to calm Ben down. Once Sheila spent an entire afternoon walking with him around the grounds, just talking and trying to get through to him.

"The sports coaches are concerned that he's lost a lot of weight," she says. I tell her I already know this; I've had a chat with the Head of Year. "And the netball coach saw him pushing himself hard in the gym, almost as if he was in a trance." She looks at me, waiting for a response.

Suddenly I'm pouring it all out. Ben isn't eating. He can't stop exercising and he's isolating himself from his friends. He's getting hysterical, flailing and shrieking, crying out like a wounded animal, banging his head against walls and getting violent. Getting him out of the door in the morning is a nightmare. Picking him up from school is even worse. Meals are a battle ground and he goes to pieces most evenings. He seems to hate school. We've taken him to the GP several times but we're just told to go away with instructions to eat sensibly and come back in a week or so.

Sheila passes me some tissues, goes to fetch the coffee and sits down to talk. "How much do you know about eating disorders?" she asks in a way that makes my blood run ice cold. It's the first time someone has echoed my own concerns.

I tell her I know virtually nothing; it's not something you think about when you have a boy. I remember there was a skeletal woman at the gym who used to punish herself on the cardio equipment. People used to whisper and stare, and ask why the management allowed it. But apart from being a "diet gone wrong", I know nothing about eating disorders. Zilch.

"I did wonder," I say slowly, hoping she'll say no, it's probably just teenage angst gone a bit too far... But instead she says, "I think you should ask your GP to get Ben referred to CAMHS".

Sheila explains that CAMHS stands for *Child and Adolescent Mental Health Services*. They're the people that deal with eating disorders in our city. No, she's never come across a boy with anorexia, but - unfortunately - it looks as if all the signs are there. Deep down I know she's right. "I'm so sorry," she says. "But the good news is that eating disorders are treatable and CAMHS are very good."

But, I ask her with mounting panic, if eating disorders are about, well, *eating*, then why the extreme behaviour and moods? The thing is, Sheila explains, eating disorders are mental illnesses just as OCD or clinical depression are mental illnesses. They don't just affect the body. After all, the brain needs fuel to function. She tells me to go back to our GP and insist on a referral right away.

"Look," she says, holding the door open for me afterwards, "Whatever the school can do... whatever I can do... don't hesitate to ask for help. Call me anytime. And if I'm not here, my deputy will be. Meanwhile I'll keep a discreet eye on Ben, and the medical centre is open to him whenever he needs a bolt-hole. Or whenever *you* do for that matter, Bev". She even gives me her mobile number in case I need to get hold of her in an emergency. It's the first of many occasions when I will feel eternally grateful to her.

Later that afternoon when Paul gets home I tell him about my visit to Sheila. "Right, that's it," he announces angrily, picking up the phone and dialling the GPs' surgery. Minutes later he has a GP on the line. He insists on an immediate referral - urgently and without delay. It's clear that Paul means business and he gets his way. Good old Paul. We spend the rest of the evening trying to come to terms with the fact that our only child probably has anorexia. Ben has a mental illness. That's difficult to grasp. But, as Paul says, by catching it early enough we should be able to get it sorted out fairly quickly. Ben's not like the woman at the gym by any stretch of the imagination. *Well not yet, at any rate,* we think to ourselves silently. We wait for CAMHS to get in touch.

BEN IS STILL COMING HOME from school with tales of how so-and-so annoyed him. Or of how he's being ignored by everyone as if he's invisible. It's become our prime topic of conversation as Ben gets increasingly agitated and upset.

One evening, following a particularly distressing meltdown, I attempt to give him a reassuring cuddle, even though my whole being wants to slap him and yell: *Stop this!! For God's sake stop this!!!*

Ben stands there rigid - unemotional, blank and numb - staring ahead into space like a zombie. "Please Ben," I plead, tears streaming down my face. "Just tell me what's wrong... Please tell me what's wrong so we can do something about it..."

"Can't you see?" he screams suddenly, making me jump out of my skin. "Whatever I say, whatever I do, I just get ignored - no-one talks to me!"

At the heart of the problem lies one boy. This boy is the cleverest boy in the year and now - it seems - the most popular, especially with the girls. The image I'm getting, from what Ben says, is of this boy surrounded by an adoring public wherever he goes. This boy revels in adoration and his admirers hang on to his every word.

Meanwhile Ben fades into the background. Everyone ignores him. He doesn't get hugs. He doesn't get admired. And this boy is often too busy sending and receiving texts from his adoring public to bother with his old friend Ben.

Worse, this boy has a six pack which attracts gasps of admiration from everyone. Or at least that's Ben's version of events.

Given different circumstances, I'd laugh it off and tell Ben not to be so ridiculous. But this is serious. Deadly serious. And I feel sorry for this boy who must have no idea of the effect his actions are having on Ben.

I'm painfully aware that Ben is exercising more than ever in a bid to get that coveted six pack so he'll be "loved" (his words) like this boy. But the more Ben exercises and the less he eats, the more weight and muscle he loses. And the more the eating disorder forces him to withdraw socially, the more impossible the task becomes. It is a vicious circle. And Ben is blind to what is happening.

BUT IT'S NOT ALL BAD NEWS. Sometimes the emerging eating disorder gives us a bit of time off. Bonfire Night - 5th November - is one such occasion. For once the weather is fine and dry, but because it's so very cold we've packed a hot picnic to take to the local fireworks display. I've baked large jacket potatoes and inserted a couple of hot sausages into each with some fried onions and BBQ sauce. (Yes, *fried* onions…) I've also taken along some of Ben's home-made gingerbread and mulled apple juice in a thermos flask, crossing my fingers that he will eat it all.

For once everyone is relatively relaxed. By now my inner ear problem has receded, too, so I feel much more like my old self. Also, to my relief, Ben eats everything without any fuss. That's what's so odd, I think to myself again. It's like Jekyll and Hyde. One moment he's relatively okay and the next he's a monster. After the fireworks the three of us make our way home along the dark suburban streets, kicking the fallen leaves as we go. Just like any other family.

But I can't totally relax. Underneath I know that the monster, demon or whatever nickname we give Ben's condition will be back, picking up where it left off and dragging him below the surface.

IT'S AGES BEFORE I can say the "A" word. *Anorexia.* For some reason the term *eating disorder* doesn't sound as serious whereas *anorexia* conjures up terrifying images in my head of skeletal people that are more like the walking dead. Or celebrities like Karen Carpenter and Lena Zavaroni who lost their fight against the condition. Or that woman at the gym.

Frightened of what this illness could do to my child, I spend a lot of time Googling for anything I can find on eating disorders. Like any condition you look up, there's so much information - some of it written by "experts", some by parents of children with eating disorders, some by the patients themselves, and most of it pretty scary.

It's also confusing. One website says this, and another says that... Then there are the sensationalist media reports featuring celebrities with eating disorders or extreme "before and after" photos of someone that's recovered from anorexia. Or someone that hasn't.

Finally there are the sinister websites written by people who are only just hanging onto the threads of their brittle lives, their bodies permanently damaged or disabled from the effects of long term starvation. What's doubly frightening is the impression I'm getting that, once ensnared, this is something that is very hard to break free from. These "hardened anorexics" are well aware they're destroying themselves, yet they seem powerless to do anything about it. A bit like a drug addict hooked on heroin - some may get clean while others never do. I'm quickly realising that anorexia isn't something you can just "snap out of" or a "diet gone too far".

If only it was this straightforward.

And still there is no sign of an appointment with CAMHS.

7

consumed

I PRINT OUT A PILE OF information that I'm convinced will scare the pants off Ben and stop him driving himself down this destructive path.

"Listen to what this woman writes," I say to him. "Her anorexia is so bad she's in a wheelchair and her internal organs are in shreds." I remind him that this is what eating disorders can do if you take them too far. I pray it's gone in and will make Ben see sense. I still can't get my head around why - even when faced with the destructive consequences... even when faced with the undisputable evidence that this kind of behaviour doesn't make you more popular or attractive - Ben doesn't seem to want to do anything about it. Or is it that he *can't* do anything about it?

I get angry. Not in front of Ben but when I'm alone. Impotently so, because I know the anger won't achieve anything. I thump the table. I kick things. I scream and shout. For the first time I'm experiencing the anger and frustration that has no solution - or, at least, no obvious solution. I feel like someone who's been thrown into a dungeon from which there's no escape.

The human instinct with a problem, even a monumental problem, is to find a solution and work towards it. Or at least that's my own personal instinct. But all you can do is attempt to scale the slimy walls knowing that you're just going to slide back down again into the darkness. I feel helpless - and hopeless.

The various help lines I stumble across don't seem to offer much hope other than emphasising the importance of getting your child treated as soon as possible. The first person accounts I send off for don't have happy endings because the author never truly recovers. At the end of the book they're still starving themselves, self-harming or whatever destructive behaviour is driving them. Apart from hoping our CAMHS appointment arrives in the post very soon, there's very little I can do. If I try to talk it through with Ben, he just blanks me or bites my head off. It's as if he's lost all his logic and rational thinking. My head is thumping. I wish to hell I could be doing something to stop the rot. Something, anything… I reach for a glass of wine.

As my panic rises, I even try visiting the local church in an attempt to find emotional support. I read about miracles in the Bible and wonder why on earth Ben can't be miraculously healed too. I feel as if I'm praying and pleading to a God that doesn't exist. And, despite being sympathetic, no-one in the church really "gets it". No-one has any idea of the agony I am going through and how I'm beginning to fear for my child's life. The thought strikes me that I'm arriving home from church more depressed than when I set off. That can't be right.

WATCHING YOUR CHILD descend into anorexia is excruciating. Many a time I wish there was a magic pill he could take and - hey presto! - the old Ben would be back. Unlike a physical illness, you can't take medication to cure it. You can't have an operation to cut it out. Worse, the wonderful, level-headed, intelligent child you've spent all these years rearing has undergone a dramatic transformation into a volatile stranger whose very sanity seems to have gone AWOL.

You feel angry. Can't he see what he's doing to himself and to us? *You feel frightened.* How long will this last? Will we ever get our boy back? *You feel frantic.* What damage is it doing to his body? Could something tip the balance and lead to him taking his own life: the dreaded "S" word that we never mention and daren't even think about?

You feel preoccupied. You can't think of anything but anorexia and what it's doing to your child. *You feel jealous.* Why is everyone else's child okay while mine isn't? *You feel guilty.* Is it something we've done as parents? Should we have picked up on it sooner?

Anorexia also makes you feel very isolated. And it's so difficult to talk to a lay person about it. To the outside world it's such a little-known, much misunderstood and even taboo condition. Living with anorexia is like living in a surreal world: a world where you pretend that everything is just fine when in reality you are falling off a cliff.

I HAVE A CHAT WITH MY sister, Alison, who has another Google around to see what she can find. She sends me a few links including one to a book called *Boys Get Anorexia Too* by Jenny Langley which I immediately send off for. When it arrives I can't put it down. For the first time I'm reading about a teenage boy who - much like Ben - develops anorexia. Also - just like Ben - he's into sport. Page after page I feel like shouting "Me too!" as I recognise the signs, symptoms and experiences; Jenny could be describing our family. Finally I've found someone else who has been through this nightmare.

To keep my spirits up, I keep going back to the end of Jenny's book; the bit where her son recovers, goes to university and begins to lead a normal life. If her family can do it, then so can we. I have no idea *how* we'll do it, mind you, but we'll damn well do it. I feel a little more optimistic, especially with the CAMHS referral underway. When we eventually hear from them, that is…

ANOTHER MELTDOWN AND another quiet session on the sofa afterwards. Ben leans his head on my shoulder, silently sobbing with despair as I tighten my grip around his shoulders as if I can fill him with some kind of healing force. If only...

"Mum, I feel so trapped!" he cries out. I can hear the desperation in his voice as he reaches out to me for help. "It's not going as I planned! It's not turning out how I thought it would!" The seductive singing of the anorexia Sirens has lured an unsuspecting Ben onto the rocks and he can't stop himself from sinking. He whispers that he just doesn't have the strength to get out of it alone. I stroke his damp, matted hair and promise to do everything in my power to help. *But what can I do?* Other than share cautionary tales about what anorexia could do to him and insist he must fight back? Damn that CAMHS appointment. When will it arrive?

Ben was to tell me much later that, by this point, his life had become little more than input and output. "I thought about food and exercise all the time. I couldn't focus on anything else, not school work, not social life, not hobbies, not anything. I couldn't even have fun, because that would be wasted time when I could be exercising. I was incredibly lonely and - ironically - the only thing that took my mind off this new loneliness was thinking about food and exercising. It was a vicious circle."

By mid-November it's as if the old Ben has been completely consumed. What is left is someone we don't recognise. Physically he's lost one quarter of his body weight. Mentally he's gone off the rails. By now I know a fair bit about the effects that starvation has on the body. But what I never get used to is the distressing behaviour - or the way that, just when you think you're seeing a chink of light at the end of the tunnel - ker-pow! - you're back to square one, fighting the demon. The revolving doors go round and round...

Also, just when you think your child has reached their lowest point, something happens that drags things even deeper. I always thought that anorexia was just about eating - or, rather, not eating - but I'm rapidly discovering that it's about so much more.

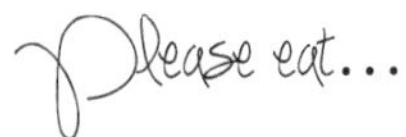

I beg, I plead, I "prove" to Ben that I can eat mountains of food without batting an eyelid. And that, if I can do it, so can he. "Look! Half a packet of biscuits! A whole box of chocolates! See, it doesn't bother me one jot - and, you know me, always on a diet, hey?" I attempt a little laugh as if this is the normal, everyday me. *Oh how relaxed I am around food; see how much I can eat without putting on an ounce of weight!*

I cry, I weep, I shout, I scream, I negotiate… but I just can't get through. He won't listen. He *can't* listen.

I am so desperate that I decide the only way I can communicate with Ben is to write him a letter. A part of me still believes that, somehow, we can snap him out of this; that he will suddenly see sense and stop this destructive behaviour. The problem is, I have no idea how. Maybe a letter will work. Maybe when he reads how terrified and upset we are he will come to his senses and stop.

Maybe… Just maybe…

So one afternoon, while waiting in the car for Ben to finish school, I carefully put pen to paper.

Dear Ben

Please read this letter. Hopefully by putting it down on paper I can get everything across without either of us getting upset or shouting at each other.

Anorexia is dangerous and needs to be stopped RIGHT NOW before it gets any worse. Getting back to a normal way of eating may take time and it probably won't be easy. But, however long it takes and no matter how hard it may seem, we want you to know that we'll be right behind you.

Your happiness and health are our Number One priority. Your dad and I want you to know that we will always be there for you, no matter how sad you feel - and we will get the very best help for you.

You know the value of healthy eating and all the reasons why you need to eat the right stuff - and enough of the right stuff - for a growing boy. This means you're much more likely to understand the massive damage this could do to your body if the anorexia gets any worse.

We love you too much to watch this happen which is why, as your loving parents, we need to step in and say "STOP! Enough is enough!" We will make serious promises to you, as our dearest son, if you make serious promises to us - and keep them.

You are more important to us than you could possibly ever imagine or even know. Please don't think there is no solution because THERE IS. Very much so. But meanwhile, ANY time you feel sad or you feel it's too hard, PLEASE talk to us - about ANYTHING. Don't bottle it up - and let us all start thinking positively now, even if that may at first, or even second, seem hard. It's not just you that's doing this alone - it's all three of us… our strong family unit. Again, I can't emphasise how much we love you and will be with you all the way through this.

Big hugs x 10 million and even more,

Mum and dad xxxxxxxxxxxxxx

I read it to Ben who listens in silence. I get the impression he wants to take action. But something tells me it's already too late. By the end of November we are all being dragged down stream so fast we can barely think. The outbursts have become more frequent, often several times a day - vicious destructive outbursts with loud screaming and tearful hysterics. It's as if Ben is having a complete mental breakdown.

IN 2012 WHEN I'M writing the draft for this book, I ask Ben to tell me more about this period.

"I realised there was a problem," he says. "I knew I needed help but I didn't like to admit it. But, to be honest, I didn't think the need was that urgent. I knew I wasn't feeling good mentally. But I was happy with my body; I didn't think it would get any worse. Being thin meant I didn't have to worry about getting fat. Yes I felt weak and generally unwell, but I just assumed it was part of being a teenager. But I admit I *was* worried about all the fuss I was creating."

He explains that he took some photographs of himself back then "which I've never told you about and would rather not show you". He goes on to say: "I was almost in awe at how thin I'd become. Yet at the same time I was terribly sad at how bad it had got. I couldn't quite believe it. But I remember looking at those photos and thinking 'This is as far as I'm going to allow myself to go'."

I HAVE A PHOTOGRAPH OF BEN which is taken in late November 2009. I've always taken lots of photos of Ben, but as he gets thinner I find it too painful. As a result this photo is one of the few I take at this stage. Ben has a big skull, and in this photo it looks out of proportion with his body. The muscles and flesh on his arms and legs have disappeared, and instead of being well-rounded and shapely, his calves have become straight. To be honest, he looks half dead.

By this time his skeletal framework is becoming more and more pronounced. Standing in his underpants I can see his shoulder blades sticking out. His hip bones and his over-large knee joints look like the kind of thing you might see on a third world famine report. His vertebrae stand out in angry bumps down his back, red raw from umpteen sit-ups as the bones rub against the fleshless skin.

The first time I see him walking around like this I feel physically sick. *Remember when those underpants were tight?* Now they hang off him, wafting around his bony thighs and sitting loosely on his protruding hip bones.

But he can't see any of this. All he sees is "fat".

His skin is dry, especially around the finger joints where it is red and itchy. His increasingly blank face has black rings around the eyes and all the fun and zest for life has been stripped from his expression. Yet, night after night, he'll sit on the sofa, rolling up his shirt to pinch the "rolls of fat" on his abs, and prodding his new "double chin".

We wait and wait to hear from CAMHS. I call the GPs' surgery to see if they know how long it will be. *Can anything be done to speed it up? No? Are you sure?* Then, on December 1st, a letter arrives in an official NHS envelope.

I can hardly contain my excitement as I rip open the envelope and unfold the letter inside.

8

bombshell

"SO," I SAY TO THE PERSON I've been asked to call at CAMHS, "When it says 'waiting list', how long are we talking about?"

"At the moment you're probably looking at around 18 to 22 weeks," comes the reply I don't want to hear.

"But my son needs to be seen urgently!" I hear the panic rising in my voice. "He's lost a quarter of his body weight, he's exercising like mad and he seems to have gone completely insane!"

"Unfortunately there's a lot of demand at the moment," she says with some sympathy. "I can't do any more than place you on the waiting list. Once an appointment for an assessment becomes available we'll write to you with a date."

"So, once he's been assessed, when does the actual treatment start?" I ask with mounting panic.

"Once they've decided what course of action to take."

"Which will be… when?"

She can't say; it's up to the assessor to decide. We will get a maximum of three assessments before they make a decision. *Three* assessments? *How long will that take?*

"Is there nothing you can do to bring an appointment forward?" I'm desperate. A quick calculation tells me it could be mid-April before we're seen. But CAMHS won't budge. There's nothing we can do but wait. I feel totally powerless. I want to scream. I get in the car and drive round to my sister's house to get it out of my system.

"Good God, he got seen faster when he broke his nose in rugby!" I say as Alison hands me a coffee. "18 to 22 weeks is around five months!" My mind quickly rewinds to where we were five months ago... June... A lot can happen in five months. "In June we didn't even know Ben was getting sick! Look how far he's gone downhill since then. Imagine what another five months could do to him? And to us? God Almighty, Ben could be *dead!*"

I think back to the days when Ben was a baby, when the NHS would pull out all the stops to ensure he developed healthily. Midwives, health visitors, baby clinics, GPs... The slightest hint of a health or growth issue and - zap, pow! - he'd be in front of a paediatrician in an instant. Like the time he appeared to be developing bow legs when he was 12 months old.

Now he's a teenager it's as if they don't care. "The crazy thing is," I cry, "he's the same human being. And this time he has an illness which could kill him. *What's not urgent about that?* I bet if he had cancer they'd fast-track him into treatment quickly enough."

I feel physically sick. Potentially five months to wait until treatment, five months during which time who knows what could happen. "And who's to say the treatment will work right away?" I say. "What if it doesn't? What if Ben spirals even further downhill?" My mind starts to go to dark places...

"Have you thought about going private?" Alison asks. "At least it'd provide a stop-gap. And hopefully it might prevent things from getting any worse. Who knows, it might even work!"

Suddenly I remember we've got some private medical insurance - a perk that comes with Paul's job. I call the insurer the moment I get home. Yes, they do cover us for mental health issues. But unfortunately it's only £500 a year. We will need to pay for any treatment over and above this. Not a problem, I say. I'd sell my soul to get my son back.

"If money's going to be an issue, we're happy to pay for some of it," Alison says when I call her back with the news. I can feel myself filling up. I want to hug that generous sister of mine.

"I've got some savings, too," I add. And I'm sure mum and dad would help, and Paul's parents too.

But I can't stop being angry. The irony is that, in a country with a free National Health Service, we're being forced to go private to rid our son of an illness which I'm quickly realising has the power to kill him.

It shouldn't happen. But it is.

THE NEXT DAY I SIT IN THE school car park waiting for Ben to finish classes drumming my fingers on the notepad where I'm making notes and adding up my savings.

Where do we find a private therapist? How do we know it will work? Paul and I are completely new to this, yet here we are facing the prospect of finding urgent life-saving treatment for our child but we don't have the first idea where to start.

The school bell rings and hordes of teenagers flock out of the building, laughing and joking, some throwing a rugby ball around while others swing on the railings. One boy kicks a football so high it lands on the sports hall roof. The Deputy Head swoops in to give him a swift telling off. Just another normal school day, I think to myself looking out from my surreal bubble.

Then Ben appears, a solitary figure, loitering far behind the others. His pale, bony appearance contrasts with the other boys. Remember the days when he'd be laughing and joking with them? Kicking a rugby ball around as they headed for the pitch on match days?

As he climbs into the car his face has a haunted look and his blank eyes are framed by dark rings. I daren't ask him how he got on at school. "Just drive," he commands in the slow, deep, dangerous tone I've come to dread. I feel the tears beginning to prick behind my eyes as I'm ordered around like a servant. Ben sits in silence all the way home, staring at nothing.

Once home, he sits in the car. I get out and open the house door, but he's still sitting in the car, still staring at nothing with cold, wide eyes. I go into the house and potter around a bit, my stress levels getting higher. Ben is still in the car and he's still staring into space.

Suddenly the car door slams and Ben crashes into the hallway and clambers up the two staircases to his attic bedroom where he slams the door. I sit on a stool in the living room, head in my hands, tissue box within reach. Is there ever a day when I don't cry?

As a family we eat our evening meals at the dining room table. We like to get together and talk about the day, without the distraction of the TV. We even eat at the table when it's just Ben and me. But with the anorexia demon at the table as well, meals have changed beyond recognition.

I'm already in a state of high anxiety wondering what the trigger will be this time. Maybe the food won't be hot enough, or there will be a danger food on his plate, or - more often than not - the portion will be too big or too small and it will throw him into confusion. Perhaps the combination of foods will be wrong. One day - for instance - I produce home-made veggie burgers in a bread bun with home-cooked oven chips. The demon doesn't like it and Ben brings his fist down on the dinner plate, smashing it and making the food splatter around. Oh hell, it dawns on me, I put breadcrumbs in the burger. Bun plus crumbs plus chips equals too many carbohydrates in one go, and - boy - am I being punished for it now.

I can always tell when things are about to erupt. Ben's face reddens, and then he quickly glances from one item to another, weighing up the situation. For a moment he's silent. Then he suddenly slams down his knife and fork, bashing his fists on the plate and sending the food flying before storming out of the room. Outside in the hallway he stamps and crashes around, thumping things and smashing his head against the wall while howling like an animal in pain. Then he hurtles up and down the hallway, banging, crashing and wailing, before disappearing up the stairs to his bedroom and slamming the door.

Meanwhile I'm left sitting at the dinner table, looking down at my food. I can't eat. I can't do anything except get annoyed at the hot tears I'm allowing to stream down my face. I sit there with my hands over my wet eyes - my head thudding - another box of tissues at hand. These days I have a box in every room.

10 or 15 minutes later Ben comes back into the room silently, almost like a sleep walker. He sits down, robotically picks up his knife and fork, rearranges whatever mess he created earlier and resumes eating in silence. I am silent, too. I daren't say anything in case it sets off the demon again. I've lost my appetite - the food tastes like cardboard. But I can't afford to leave any food on my plate when I'm eating with my anorexic son.

The rest of the evening is a mix of violent tears, hysterics and more of the long drawn out, low-pitched animal wails. I didn't know it was possible for human beings to make a sound like this. The closest, I think, was the guttural, almost primeval noise I made when I was in labour with Ben.

I attempt to talk things through with him. Sometimes it works and sometimes it doesn't. If it doesn't, then the scene will carry on well into the night. But I know that whatever I say - or whatever positive action Ben may agree to - everything will be forgotten the next day. It isn't that he doesn't want to keep his promises; he just *can't*. The demon won't let him.

THE NEXT TIME I GET a free moment away from Ben - that brief period between getting him off to school and receiving the first communication of the day from Sheila or from Ben - I begin my search for a private therapist. Blimey, I think, this is going to be even harder than I thought. I'm stunned at the sheer variety of different therapists and approaches used to treat eating disorders. Psychiatrists, psychologists, counsellors, new age therapists, hypnotherapists, therapists that only treat adults and a bundle of acronyms as long as my arm: CBT, NLP, TFT, DBT…

Oh - and because I want to claim on our health insurance - I have to get a GP's referral. The therapist also has to be on their "approved" list. I can't choose just any Dr Tom, Dick or Harry.

The thing is, I still have no idea where to start. And what if - in my ignorance - I spend all our cash on a treatment that doesn't work? But it's not just about the money; the treatment we choose *has* to work. Period.

Over the next few days I begin an intensive cramming session on anorexia. I send off for books, call helplines, scour the internet for information and spend a lot of time talking about eating disorders with the school nurse. But even then I can't help but feel I'm just scratching the surface. Basically I haven't a clue what kind of treatment Ben needs or where we will find it. Or, when we do eventually find it, how that treatment will work. How long, I wonder, does it take to talk someone out of their anorexia and get them to eat?

Heck, I don't even know the difference between a psychiatrist and a psychologist. How on earth can I expect to make an informed decision about which life-saving treatment is best for my son?

9

going private

I DECIDE TO START AT THE top and go for a private psychiatrist. Psychiatrists seem to be the most expensive so, logic implies, their treatment must be the most effective. This means Ben will get better faster. Or at least that's the way my mind is working in the run up to Christmas in 2009. Eventually I find a psychiatrist that can see us over the busy festive season.

Friday afternoon sees us sitting opposite a rather stern, smartly dressed gentleman as the clock ticks away on the first £250 of our insurance money. But, after asking a lot of questions, it appears he'll simply be supervising the treatment. He hands me a list of suitable therapists to contact - the people that will do the real work. "Then, in a few weeks' time, you can come back and tell me how you got on." *Not at £250 a shot, we won't*, I mutter under my breath. I take the expensive list home.

Only one of the therapists is available before New Year: Karen, a therapist specialising in CBT (Cognitive Behavioural Therapy). This, I discover, is a talking therapy widely used to help people with mental health problems including eating disorders. The idea is that, through talking, a CBT practitioner can help the patient identify and change extreme thinking and behaviour. Or at least that's what the internet says as I do a quick CBT cramming session.

"But I must warn you - it's not going to be a quick fix," Karen explains when I call her. "To be honest Ben needs to be treated by a team of people - like CAMHS. I only do CBT. But I'll see what I can do."

She doesn't sound very positive, I think, wondering if we're wasting our time and money. But I guess it's better than nothing and by now I am desperate.

OCCASIONALLY WE SEE a glimpse of something that almost resembles the old Ben. He'll calm down from the latest rage and sit with his head on my shoulder, clinging onto my hand as if I'm a lifebuoy in a stormy sea. But it's always short-lived. Before long the demon is back, spitting venom, getting violent and shrieking at me to f*ck off. When you're only 5ft 3 and female it's not easy to restrain a teenage boy. I've no idea where stick-thin Ben gets his strength from.

Working out our weekly menus is becoming harder than ever. By now we're limited to a minuscule range of meals, each containing ingredients which I know Ben will eat without too much fuss. Ben's policing of the kitchen is also getting worse. Often I'll find him checking there's no contraband in the fridge, freezer or larder. Everything has to be zero fat and if an extra-light version is available then we have to buy that. One day he tips all the cheese into the trash bin because, it appears, we're not allowed to eat cheese any more. I stand there aghast.

Woe betides me if I attempt to fry anything. Even frying a chopped onion in a tablespoon of oil is a criminal offence. *Why fry when you can dry-fry?* The slightest globule of oil is described as "swimming in fat" and results in violent refusals to eat. When you've just cooked a meal that your child refuses to eat, what can you do? If it was a normal teenager you'd tell them that it's either this or nothing. But with a teenager with anorexia you can't; you know they have to eat. Sometimes I end up cooking a brand new meal - or, on the occasions when I've reached the end of my tether and have to get out of the kitchen before I smash the place to pieces, we'll go out to eat. Not a great experience, as you can imagine, when your child has anorexia, but I figure there'll be something on the menu he'll eat, even if it's only a salad (dressing-free, of course).

New recipes are risky. I take a sharp intake of breath as I remember the day when I foolishly decided to cook smoked mackerel burgers. *Was I aware of how much fat there is in mackerel?* All day long thoughts of "fat-laden" mackerel buzzed around Ben's head. I knew because he kept texting me about it. By the time he arrived home he was in a terrible state.

At meal times our portions have to be identical. Absurdly I find myself weighing them out in front of Ben to prove there isn't a nano gram more on his plate than on ours. If there is he'll throw a wobbly - or remove food from his plate and deposit it on mine. "I've got loads more than you, mum," he'll say accusingly.

I used to love cooking and now I loathe it. From the moment I walk into the hated kitchen I'm in a state of high anxiety. The slightest creak on the staircase and I'll throw the ("extra lean") minced beef, tomatoes or whatever into the chopped onion which I've dared to fry in oil. I'll stir vigorously to remove any sign of oil and then stir it again just to make sure. And all the time I pretend to be acting normally. Sometimes I even find myself nervously singing songs in a bid to distract Ben from what's going on in the kitchen. With Christmas just around the corner I sing *Winter Wonderland* over and over again until I'm sick to death of it. *See, I am so H-A-P-P-Y and R-E-L-A-X-E-D.*

As a mother it has always been my job to feed my child, and my son has a lifelong history of demolishing food as if it's going out of fashion. Before the anorexia he'd hoover up every single morsel - and demand more - while I'd look on with indulgent satisfaction. My son could eat for England. Yet now the thought of feeding him puts the fear of God into me. One false move and - ker-pow! - the demon erupts. I live in dread of Ben walking into the kitchen to find me adding an extra tablespoon of oil to the pot.

A lay person might say: "For God's sake, just make him eat. To hell with the repercussions; you're his parents!"

But it's almost impossible to describe the ice cold fear you have of the demon: the thing that's inside Ben which, without much provocation, could make him take his own life rather than eat. By this time suicide is a constant worry. I feel as if we're living on a perpetual knife-edge

I find myself hiding contraband like cheese, ground almonds and so on in strange places, ready to slip into the mix as soon as Ben is upstairs, my body ramrod straight with tension in case I'm found out - frantically tasting the food to make sure the extra ingredients aren't detectable. If in doubt, I don't add anything. The sheer blind terror I feel at times like these is beyond description. Yet at the same time I can't help but notice the absurdity of it all. Here we have a teenage boy who, like most teenage boys, should be eating his parents out of house and home. Yet I'm terrified of a small chunk of cheese.

Only the other week a mother was laughing about how her ravenous teenage son would arrive home from school, get out the bread, slather on the butter and proceed to systematically clear the contents of the fridge. Her son, she exclaimed, had a huge breakfast every day and then you'll never guess what he did next? He stopped to pick up a friend on the way to school and had a second breakfast there!

It seems ludicrous that here am I, the parent of a teenage boy the same age, my hand trembling with fear as I get some grated butter out of the freezer, tip some of it out and stir it into the rice pudding, all the time listening to make sure Ben isn't coming back downstairs. Then I hide the butter at the back of the freezer again. No it isn't ludicrous; it is heart-breaking. *How the hell did my son end up like this?* I long for him to rush into the house after school, cram calorific snacks into his mouth and still be ravenous by suppertime. I wouldn't give a damn about how much my food shopping cost me; I'd get a second mortgage if necessary. If only my son would eat…

A couple of years later this all comes out into the open as I'm reading this manuscript to Ben. "You deceived me!" he interrupts as I try to explain why I "tweaked" the food occasionally.

"Yes, I admit I did add extra calories wherever I could," I respond. "Heck, Ben, you were falling off a cliff - I was fighting to save your life. I'd have done anything to save you. Any mother would do it. *You'd* do it if you were a parent, I guarantee it."

"But I thought I could trust you."

"You could and can trust me, Ben, and you know that. But back then, while you were sliding into goodness only knows where, I was terrified the eating disorder would destroy you. I couldn't just sit back and do nothing."

ONE DAY I DECIDE TO STRIP all the grocery shopping of its packaging so Ben can't home in on the nutritional labels or tell if it's high fat, low fat or no fat. I also scribble out the calories and fat content from recipes. Out of sight, I reason, means out of mind. But I haven't figured on Ben knowing every individual calorific value off by heart. Ben, who's always been pretty weak at maths, is a genius when it comes to adding up calories in his head and working out fat content.

I even toy with the idea of swapping foods around - of buying standard cheese instead of fat-reduced cheese and putting it in a low fat wrapper, or substituting zero fat yoghurt for full-fat.

Crazy scenarios like me standing in the supermarket car park decanting higher fat products into zero fat containers, then rushing to the trash bin to get rid of the evidence; even swapping the labels around on milk cartons.

Absurdly, I worry Ben will appear out of nowhere and I'll be found out. I begin to know where all the trash bins are located on the way to school. Ping! In goes another cheese wrapper or yoghurt pot.

I hate the person who invented those nutritional wheels on food packaging - the information that's supposed to alert everyone to "healthy eating". I suspect many people ignore them. But not teenagers with anorexia; people like Ben are drawn to nutritional information like bees to a honeypot.

I also hate those people that are cramming our supermarket shelves with diet products. None of this stuff existed when I was Ben's age. Yet, curiously, we have a bigger problem with obesity than ever. Something is seriously wrong. I want to put skull and crossbones stickers on every "light", "lite", "extra-lite", "skimmed", "fat reduced", "diet", "healthy" and "low calorie" product there is. Warning: *keep away from your anorexic child...*

Once upon a time recipes were written without any nutritional breakdown. You'd just lob everything into the pot, cook it and eat it - just as it's been done since the world began.

But, in today's obesity-obsessed and oh-so-H-E-A-L-T-H-Y 21st century, everything has to be measured out accurately and subdivided into calories, umpteen different kinds of fats and other nutrients, all of which are meticulously listed below each recipe. It's like manna from heaven to the anorexia demon.

I catch Ben going through the recipes, ticking all the "safe" meals to "help me out". He crosses out all the added fats and other "baddies", suggesting "healthier" alternatives and writing comments about why we don't need "that much" cheese or meat. He puts a huge "X" through any unsuitable recipes. The more vigorous the "X" the higher the calorie and fat content.

"You're not on a diet, Ben!" I sigh for the umpteenth time. I am wasting my breath.

I remove a stack of Good Food and Delicious magazines from the kitchen cupboard to a bookcase in my bedroom and dig out all those old recipe books, the ones without "healthy" nutritional information.

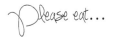

But, by now, Ben can add up the calories and fats in a recipe just by looking at it.

BEN ISN'T ENTHUSIASTIC ABOUT seeing Karen, the private CBT therapist. He doesn't want treatment; he doesn't feel he needs treatment. Karen makes it clear that we won't get anywhere unless Ben agrees to work with her. Nothing in Ben's expression or body language indicates that he has any intention of working with her, or with anyone. He just sits there silently, black rings under his eyes, painfully thin and waif-like in the pyjama pants he's been wearing for the yoga sessions he does after school. He doesn't want to be there.

Over three or four sessions Karen does her level best to get through to Ben, but he's not reacting or listening. But, to his credit, he does some of the "homework" she sets him, like making a daily list of positive things that have happened in order to raise his mood. But he soon gives up. "It's been a sh*t day so I've nothing positive to write," he says again and again, leaving the list untouched.

Despite all her good intentions, I can't help feeling that our sessions with Karen are like trying to plug the hole in the Titanic with cotton wool. I have no idea how talking is supposed to make Ben change his mind and regain all the lost weight. Or how long it will take. Or how terribly thin he will have to get before it bears fruit.

I feel as if we're floating adrift in a huge ocean with no land in sight. The escalating eating disorder has transformed my son beyond all recognition - yet all pleas to speed up our CAMHS appointment are falling on deaf ears. I am powerless to get my son the treatment I believe he so urgently needs and which, in a country with a free National Health Service, he should be entitled to.

10

admiring cakes

A FEW WEEKS BEFORE CHRISTMAS the three of us do some last-minute Christmas shopping in Manchester's Trafford Centre. The demon is thankfully absent and Ben is back to his normal self. Or at least the normal self we're getting used to - the Ben that automatically goes for the diet or low calorie option when it comes to choosing a take-out lunch from Boots or Marks & Spencer.

Ben you're not on a diet, I want to yell…

But we manage to shop, have a laugh and eat. We're (almost) like any other family getting excited by all the festive lights and sparkle. A famous celebrity is signing his latest book and the place is milling with teenage girls and their mothers. I watch them form a long queue outside the bookstore. My eyes move along the line. Here we have a full range of physiques from the big to the positively skinny. Too skinny, I worry…

"I can't be bothered to cook tonight," I say as we leave, exhausted, late in the afternoon. I suggest we go to Pizza Express. Risky, I know, but I'm completely shopped-out.

So we do. And we eat pizzas, just like any other family. No-one would ever guess there's anything amiss. Unless, of course, they could see into my mind which, as ever, is coiled up like a spring ready for the demon to strike. So far the demon has left us alone in public. So far…

Ben orders a pizza. So far so good. And he eats it. So far even better. Then the waitress asks if we'd like to see the dessert menu. I wait for Ben to decline, but - to my surprise - he orders a chocolate fudge sundae and proceeds to eat every bit. I watch with astonishment as he spoons the sticky, sickly chocolate toffee concoction into his mouth. I wonder what's going on inside his head.

"At this stage I wanted to prove I could conquer the illness without treatment," he tells me years later. "But oh my God did the anorexia beat me up afterwards for eating that huge pizza and pudding!"

IT'S BEN'S PRE-BIRTHDAY party and sleepover a week before Christmas, just like last year. Only it isn't just like last year. The usual suspects are there, but this time they're unusually quiet. I take a peek into Ben's bedroom where the boys are silently playing computer games. *Is it my imagination or could you cut the atmosphere with a knife?* One boy complains of feeling unwell, so his mum drives over to pick him up. At bedtime, it's the first time in the history of Ben's sleepovers that I haven't had to bash on the door and tell them to be quiet. The house is completely silent.

Just after midnight a loud crash wakes us with a start.

Paul and I rush onto the landing. Ben is charging down the two flights of stairs, howling like a wounded animal and hurtling towards the living room door. We fly downstairs. He's in a terrible state: weeping and almost hyperventilating. "Ben! Stop it!" Paul shouts, grabbing Ben's fists which he's thumping against the living room door. It turns out that one of his friends was irritating him and Ben flipped. Meanwhile all is unnaturally silent upstairs.

The next morning a subdued group of boys makes their way downstairs for breakfast, making polite conversation, trying to pretend that the previous night didn't happen.

It's a relief when their parents collect them. I can sense the mums and dads looking critically at Ben - and I can't resist looking at their sons as they come downstairs. Big, burly boys followed by a skinny, waif-like Ben. It's a long time since the parents have seen Ben and I can't help wondering what they're thinking.

ON THE SUNDAY BEFORE Christmas we go to a carol service. An abandoned church is being brought back to life and this is the first service that's been held there for decades. Everyone has been told to wrap up warm because there's no heating in the semi-derelict building and it's snowing heavily outside.

There is no organ - just a gaping hole where it used to be, cordoned off with some hazard tape. Plaster is peeling off the damp walls and some of the stained glass has been vandalised. There's no lighting in the dark interior, just a few twinkling fairy lights which someone has managed to rig up as well as dozens of candles.

It is freezing. So cold, you can see your breath. Colder than anyone, I suspect, is Ben, wrapped up in layer upon layer of clothing, his nose red and his skin pale, almost translucent in the candlelight.

I'm aware of him staring at the gap where the long-removed altar once stood, a desperate look on his face. As the choir sings carols, I can see tears welling up in his eyes - and, after the service, he walks over to a table by the old stone font and picks up some leaflets and a St Mark's gospel. I can almost physically feel him reaching out for help. I fantasize about a bolt of heavenly healing streaking through the vaulted gothic roof and into Ben's soul.

But, of course, nothing happens and we leave the atmospheric church without anyone being any the wiser that our son so desperately needs help.

COOKING IS A RISKY BUSINESS, especially with Christmas drawing closer. But Ben can't keep out of the kitchen. There he is, apron on, ready to cook another "healthy" version of something-or-other. It only takes one thing to go wrong and - zap! - the demon swoops in. Earlier that afternoon I'd heard a tell-tale crash coming from the kitchen accompanied by an almost primeval howl of "NOOOOOOOOO!" followed by "Sh*t! Sh*t! Sh*t!" Then the sound of something being thrown or slammed onto the work surface. Ben stamped his feet with an almighty force before fleeing upstairs yelling. The (fat free) cake he'd been baking was too dry.

My cooking has to be perfect, too. I feel as if I'm appearing on a hellish version of TV's Masterchef. If I fail to make the grade, even by a minuscule bit, the demon will blow a fuse. By Christmas I've got to the stage where I'm in mortal dread of setting it off. The trouble is the demon can spot the kind of imperfection that's undetectable to the naked eye - so I never know whether I've slipped up until it's too late. Too hot, too cold, too much, too dry, too soggy, too bland, too oily…

Despite my better judgement, I let Ben make some ginger cookies to decorate the Christmas tree: angels, stars, Christmas trees, holly leaves and Santas, each with satin red ribbon threaded through a hole made by a drinking straw. Predictably he sets about making a "healthy" version, eliminating all the fat and reducing the sugar content. Unusually he doesn't fly off the handle when - surprise, surprise - the cookies are tasteless and rock hard. Still, at least they look festive hanging on the Christmas tree with their pretty red ribbons.

A couple of days before Christmas and it's Ben's 16th birthday. We've been to the cinema with my sister followed by a surprisingly angst-free curry (Alison has deliberately chosen a "healthy" Indian restaurant to appease the demon).

Towards the end of the meal the snow begins to fall thick and fast, and eventually the car gets stuck in a drift. We make our way back to the house on foot, trudging up the middle of the silent street past house upon house of twinkling Christmas lights.

Once home, Paul coaxes the embers in the grate back to life, we switch on the tree lights and I light some scented candles. For a brief moment I'm transported into a magical Christmas wonderland of childhood memories. Santa leaving a stocking full of toys with some chocolate coins, and an apple and orange in the toe… My dad reading Hans Christian Andersen stories in front of the coal fire by candlelight…

Ben's blank look jolts me back to the present. "I just don't feel Christmassy," he says again. Ben's mind is completely numb. It's as if he's been anesthetised.

To be honest I couldn't give a damn about Christmas, either - me who usually goes over the top with decorations covering every surface in the house, dozens of fairy lights and enough food and drink to feed an army.

It's the first year I haven't sent any Christmas cards. I just don't feel like it. Thankfully my sister has offered to cook Christmas dinner because, frankly, if it was left up to me I wouldn't bother.

On Christmas Eve I'm sitting on the sofa thinking about parents everywhere who, at Christmas, want more than anything to get their "little boy" or "little girl" back, whether it's anorexia, drugs, runaways, gangs, crime, drinks, going off the rails or worse.

I watch Paul and Ben building a snow Santa outside the house. Our neighbours trot across the road to admire it, unaware of the trauma that's going on in our lives.

Just moments later we're going through another crisis as Ben explodes in the kitchen over some calorie or food issue, I can't remember what. But I do remember sobbing that "I just want my little boy back" over and over again while *Carols from Kings* washes over my head on the radio.

Curiously, on Christmas Day, despite the worsening anorexia, Ben eats a full Christmas dinner without much complaint. The demon has given us another day off. Just one day, mind you. By Boxing Day the demon is well and truly back. And the next day when we go for a walk in the Derbyshire Peaks. Ben unnecessarily charges up and down the steep hill, and then up and down again, as if on a military training exercise, as the demon pushes him to exercise off the festive "excesses". But, to his credit, he orders a beanburger when we stop off at a café for lunch.

WINTER 2009/10 IS THE winter of the Big Freeze, the year the lake in our local park freezes solid. Ben and I trudge through the snowy wooded gorge towards the frozen lake and the ruins of what was once a stately home. Our walk gives us the opportunity to talk.

Talking like this is a little more successful than trying to talk at home. It's not so confrontational. Yet I still feel as if I'm flogging a dead horse. No matter what I say, it falls on deaf ears. Ben is unable to see logic or reason. He will argue that black is white until he is blue in the face.

Actually, looking at Ben standing shivering by a ruined stone archway, it really does look as if he's blue in the face. His illness means he feels the cold more than most people so he's wrapped up warm against the freezing temperatures. But I'm painfully aware that beneath the chunky sweater, jacket, hat, scarf and gloves is an increasingly emaciated body. Yet he can't see this. *Or can he?* I'm not sure, because although he now admits that something is wrong, he still sees fat where there isn't any.

Another aspect of his illness becomes starkly clear as we stop off at a café for a hot drink (black coffee for Ben, naturally…). There, in the display cabinet, are dozens of cakes and bakes: chocolate fudge cake, carrot cake, millionaire's shortbread, coffee and walnut gateau… Ben is drawn to these like a magnet. Not to eat them, but to admire them, as you or I might admire works of art hanging in a gallery. A girl comes over to take his order and gives him an odd look when he shakes his head but continues to stare… He moves to where I'm sitting. "Mum, you have to see this cake, it's amazing!" and attempts to drag me over to "admire" the display.

I refuse.

There we are, during the festive season, living in the Western World where food is abundantly available - almost obscenely so in this café full of cakes - yet my son is starving himself. Or, rather, the anorexia is starving him. Fortunately for the wildfowl on the lake, someone's broken a large section of ice so they can swim around, fighting for the chunks of bread being tossed into the water by young families.

At least they're enjoying their food.

SHORTLY AFTER NEW YEAR we resume our sessions with Karen. I stand in the kitchen talking to her on the phone. "He's only been back at school a couple of days and already things are deteriorating." I tell her that he's depressed, feels numb, doesn't want to talk to his friends and can't stop thinking about food. "And he thinks he's getting fat. To be honest, I don't think I can cope with much more - and I know Paul can't." I hate seeing my big burly husband breaking down in tears.

Karen takes it seriously. "Look," she says, "If you like I'll write to CAMHS and ask if Ben's referral can be speeded up". I remember she said she used to work for one of the CAMHS teams in our city. "But if he loses any more weight - or starts to lose it quickly - then please promise me you'll get in touch with your GP again."

Then, at the end of January, something unexpected happens which abruptly ends our sessions with Karen.

11

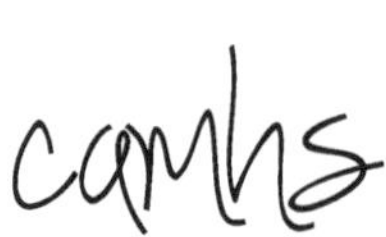

IN LATE JANUARY we finally get the long-awaited letter from CAMHS with the date of our first assessment - 16th February - much sooner than the April appointment we'd been led to expect.

But, in the event, we never get there.

A few days later, Ben is taken into hospital with the slow pulse rate described at the beginning of this book: the dash to the first hospital followed by the decision to move him by ambulance to the specialist cardio unit in the city's other main hospital.

I arrive to discover Ben undergoing more scans and tests. He is also hooked up to another machine and has an intravenous line inserted into a vein in his hand. A worried Paul arrives and I quickly take him to one side to explain what's been going on. Then, a bit later, an orderly brings in an early evening meal.

"Sorry but you arrived too late to choose from the menu," she apologises to Ben. "I hope this is okay." She deposits an unappetising plate of chicken, over-boiled vegetables and watery gravy in front of him. Not surprisingly, Ben ignores it. In a panic I have visions of wheeling in cauldrons of home-cooked food to keep him from starving. But, for tonight because - thank God - he is hungry, we'll have to settle for whatever the hospital shop has on sale. As I take the lift to the ground floor I'm struck by the absurdity of it all. There is my son, upstairs on the ward, wired up to cardio machines and undergoing a host of frightening tests - yet here am I, heading for the hospital shop, more concerned about selecting the right kind of sandwich. Sometimes living with this illness can seem like a theatrical farce or one of those hilarious silent movies where everyone is dashing around like crazy. Only this screenplay isn't hilarious; it's terrifying.

I choose a sandwich carefully, finally going for a tuna salad which I hope and pray he will eat. I also select a fruit salad, some dried fruit and a banana. *Ben, please eat it...*

"Ben has anorexia," I explain back on the ward as someone removes the untouched chicken supper. I want them to "get it", to urgently react by sending in a specialist *SWAT* team armed with mountains of life-giving food which they'll get Ben to eat. This is a hospital after all, damn it. But instead they look at me blankly. I have a sneaking suspicion they know even less about eating disorders than I do. This seems odd because already I'm aware that anorexia can affect the heart. After all, Ben's lost most of the visible muscle on his body so goodness only knows what the illness is doing to that hidden muscle: the heart.

Meanwhile half of me panics with visions of cardiac arrests, heart transplants and worse. The other half thinks, well if they're allowing him to eat then they can't be thinking of operating. And he's at *this* end of the ward and - thankfully - not *that* end (the emergency end). Also, he's not seeing the consultant until the morning; if it was critical he'd be seeing him now. Things like that...

Unfortunately at this stage the doctors are unable to say what is wrong. *Why does no-one seem overly interested in his anorexia?* My blood goes cold again. I simply have to accept that they're the professionals; they know what they are doing. Or at least I hope they do.

As Ben is taken downstairs for further tests Paul and I take a break and head for a café in the local shopping centre. Paul places the chicken and bacon sandwich that I don't feel like eating in front of me. "With any luck this'll shock Ben into seeing what he's doing to himself. Hopefully it'll give him the wakeup call he needs."

I hope and pray so, vaguely aware of people buzzing around us on the way home from work, others going out for the evening; people laughing and chatting, some probably the same age as Ben, en route to a movie in the cinema upstairs.

Later that evening Paul and I leave the hospital for home. We're exhausted. Neither of us gets a good night's sleep. I'm up at 4am, head hurting, half wondering if I'll receive an emergency phone call. By 8am we're back at the hospital.

"Thankfully," the consultant tells us when he does his rounds, "Ben's heart has stabilised." It's still beating slowly, but not slowly enough to keep him in hospital for another day - and the various tests haven't showed up anything sinister. It's the first time we've met the consultant and we're desperate to know if this problem is going to reoccur. After all, it's our child's heart we are talking about and he only has one heart.

"We often find that athletes have slow pulse rates," he says, repeating what the doctor said at the first hospital. "I understand Ben is very sporty, so - in the absence of any other reason why his pulse is slow - I suspect this might be the cause."

"Ben has anorexia," I say again. "He's had anorexia since the summer. Yes he does a lot of sport, but the main problem is that he's not eating properly and has lost an awful lot of weight and muscle."

"Well," says the consultant to Ben, "If you ever feel strange again you must promise me you'll come straight back". Fat chance of Ben doing that, I think.

On the way back to the car Ben surprises us by wanting to stop off for something to eat. "I'm starving!" he exclaims, ordering a hefty-looking bagel and proceeding to devour it hungrily.

A couple of years later he tells me this is because he wanted to prove that he could conquer the illness, without any outside help - and also because he wanted to cheer us all up. "Being in hospital put the fear of God into me; I didn't want a repeat."

WITHIN MINUTES OF ARRIVING home I call CAMHS. I tell the person who answers the phone that Ben needs to be seen right away. Not in two weeks' time, but *now*... urgently. I tell them about the heart scare. I say he's lost one quarter of his bodyweight since the summer. I describe the rages. I leave nothing out.

The person says she'll get someone to call me back.

A few moments later the phone rings. It's a consultant psychiatrist called Sarah. "Would you like to bring Ben in to see us at 9 o'clock on Monday?" she says to my amazement and relief. So - four months after I first took Ben to see our GP - we are sitting in front of Sarah and a nursing specialist called Linda.

MY FIRST IMPRESSION OF THE CAMHS unit isn't a good one. It's a small shabby building located in one of our city's most deprived areas, surrounded by run down high-rise council housing, litter-infested wasteland and dodgy-looking gangs of youths. It's the kind of area where you worry about leaving your car or walking after dark.

We sit in the waiting area which looks almost as cheerless as the exterior: high ceilings and shiny, windowless institutional walls. A radio plays in the background, presumably in an attempt to make the room feel welcoming. I glance at the notice warning that no violence or abusive behaviour will be tolerated. I later discover this building used to be a 19th century workhouse.

There's no-one else in the waiting area except me, Ben and Paul - until a smiling Sarah and Linda arrive on the scene armed with files and clipboards. Ben is taken into an ante-room to be weighed while Paul and I are directed into a featureless consulting room. Sarah apologises that the building isn't more welcoming. We sit down - the three of us opposite the two of them - with an ugly formica coffee table in between.

I notice a box of tissues on the table. *They expect tears.* There's a clock on the wall above Sarah's head. I will get to know this clock intimately over the following months, willing the hands to move slower as they creep further and further towards the end of our weekly 60 minutes.

The rusting steel-framed frosted glass window doesn't fit and, on this early February morning, a cold draught blows across the thickly painted radiator to the cork noticeboard with its faded pictures. Outside - above the frosted pane of glass - I can see a high wall with patchy flaking render and over that the grey concrete stairs of some high rise flats. It's noisy, with the sound of vehicles and people using this route as an exit from the main hospital or as a place to smoke. Sometimes we have to raise our voices just to be heard.

Nothing in this dismal room will change in the two years we spend with CAMHS. With its peeling paint, rounded institutional door frames and tall ceiling it isn't unlike the kind of cheerless room you'd expect in a 19th century mental institution. But, I think to myself, I mustn't judge a book by its cover.

Sarah leans forward in her chair. "So how's the pulse rate behaving?" she asks with concern. I say I'm not really sure, but I'm keeping an eye on it - timing it against my watch. So far it's still low, but not as low as it was. I explain that I'm worried sick that the problem might re-occur. I tell her that Ben has lost one quarter of his bodyweight since July and I'm terrified of where this is going. I can hear the pitch of my voice getting higher and faster as panic sets in. Meanwhile Sarah and Linda sit there, calmly, listening to what I have to say.

Red tape means there are lots of formalities, like form filling, signatures and so on. "Just get to the bit where you make him well," I want to yell at them as my anxiety levels rise. "Stuff the paperwork!"

Sarah explains that we'll be seeing them once a week for a 60-minute session - and Alice, a dietician, once every three weeks.

Sometimes we'll meet together as a family and at other times Ben will be seen alone by either Sarah or Linda - or both. Really and truly it's impossible to say exactly what will happen or how long the treatment will take. It's more a case of playing it by ear, experimenting and seeing how things turn out.

Experimenting? I don't know if I like the sound of that. But - despite my mounting panic - I remind myself that it's not like a physical illness. You can't prescribe a course of medication and the patient recovers in a week. I get the feeling we're going to be coming here for some time.

I take a deep breath and try to calm myself down, telling myself that we're finally with the experts. They will know what to do and how to do it. Suddenly I feel safer. We're the shipwrecked boat and they're the air-sea rescue team hovering overhead. I eagerly wait for them to hoist us from the sinking ship.

A relaxed and genial Sarah asks more questions while Linda continues to scribble notes. We sign more forms and nod our heads as the legalities are explained to us. Then in the blink of an eye the assessment is over. "No!" I want to scream. "We need more time!" Absurdly I'm convinced that the more time we spend with Sarah and Linda, the faster Ben will recover. I want them to do a cramming session, military boot camp style. Like the Weight Loss Camp that takes over the school every summer where, in theory, obese teenagers arrive for an intensive six weeks and depart slim and healthy. Problem solved.

But, far from being winched into the helicopter and flown to safety, nothing has changed. Back home life carries on as normal. Or at least the new "normal" we're reluctantly getting used to.

Seven days later we're back in that shabby room for a second assessment, listening to Sarah while Linda takes notes. Is this when they make him eat, I wonder? Where they wave a magic wand and - hey presto - via some magical persuasive technique Ben agrees to cooperate and we all live happily ever after?

I've just finished a book that insists you feed your anorexic teenager with three large meals and three snacks a day. Custard, sponge puddings, ice cream, jam, biscuits, cakes, burgers, chips, butter, cream... the more calorific and fat-laden the better. Yet nowhere in this book does it say *how* you're supposed to get the food into your child. So far I've failed to get most normal foods into my son. I haven't a hope in hell of getting him to eat steamed puddings, butter and cream. I can only assume that CAMHS will show me how to do it. Soon. Very soon. Impatiently I wait for them to get onto the subject of food.

In the end I interrupt. "Will you be putting together an eating plan for Ben?"

Linda rummages in her briefcase and digs out a sheet of paper. "This is the kind of thing we use," she says, handing me some photocopied sheets stapled together. Like the book, this eating plan expects the patient to eat three meals and three snacks a day, measured in 10 inch plate sizes and 250ml cups. "How many calories should he have in a day?" I ask.

"We prefer not to count calories. We deal in portion sizes." The sheet describes what a "portion" is.

Yet again I am faced with a long list of impossible foods in unworkable quantities. Unworkable for us, at any rate. Jam or custard doughnut? Sponge, pie or crumble with custard or ice cream? Who are they kidding?

Nevertheless I take the sheet away with me, determined to have a go. I stop off at the supermarket and grab a large trolley. I push it around the aisles zealously grabbing peanut butter, scotch pancakes, cheese, yoghurt, cookies, bread, bacon, jam, smoothies, full-fat milk... I am a mother on a mission; I can feel the adrenalin pumping through my system. It's like one of those TV game shows where you have just seconds to pack as much food as possible into your trolley.

It's almost as if, by the very action of cramming my trolley with calorie-laden goodies, I am pumping the lifeblood back into my son. Meanwhile Ben trails behind me with one of his *I don't know why you're bothering* looks. *No way will I eat any of this.*

And of course he doesn't.

But, hopefully, at our next session with CAMHS I will be shown how to roll out the eating plan successfully.

12

the eating plan

FROM THE START, I am hell-bent on getting this eating plan to work. The eating plan that will get my son well. *Eating Plan 6* it says at the top of the page. I wonder how it differs from numbers 1, 2, 3, 4 and 5… There's also a sheet where I can note down what Ben eats and when, and any compensatory behaviours. I begin to make notes.

But almost immediately I have to tweak it and ditch the idea of butter, potato crisps, sponge puddings, custard, chocolate bars and scones. After all, I can't clamp open his mouth and force-feed him. I can't hold him down and make him sit there until he's eaten every calorific, fatty bit. This is a teenage boy we're talking about; someone who - even in his skinny state - is taller and stronger than me. So, if I want to get *Eating Plan 6* to work I'm going to have to alter it. Until someone shows me how to get all these doughnuts, Mars Bars and crumbles into my child.

Portion sizes don't work, either. They might work if I was feeding him with pie, cheese and sponge puddings. But they won't work with the kind of low calorie, low fat foods Ben insists on eating. A plateful of pasta with an oil-free sauce made from extra lean mince is not the same as a plateful of creamy, buttery spaghetti carbonara. Nor is a butter-free slice of diet toast the same as the jam or custard filled doughnut which *Eating Plan 6* suggests he has for a snack. For the time being, at any rate, I'm going to have to focus on getting the right amount of food into him which is going to mean counting calories.

The trouble is - I don't know what "the right amount" is. I can only guess, based on what the internet says a 16 year old growing boy needs, and then add a bit more to ensure he gains weight. Nevertheless I am determined to get some food into him. We'll cross the dreaded fats bridge when we come to it.

BREAKFAST ON DAY ONE of the eating plan is relatively successful. But the rest of the day is trickier: snacks, juices, smoothies, sandwich lunch, dessert, evening meal, another dessert and another snack. I feel as if I'm shovelling food into Ben until he can't eat any more.

The demon doesn't like it and it's about to make sure I know it. The next day - Saturday - Ben and I go shopping in the city centre. The plan is to pick up some lunch while we're there.

Ben's always liked Pret, a café that makes its own imaginative sandwiches, salads and soups. But seconds into the busy café and I realise I've made the wrong decision. He stares miserably at all the sandwiches, baguettes and salads in the large display cabinet.

"Go on, choose one," I say a little too brightly. "How about this? Or this one? That looks nice." I sense my stress levels rising. I pretend to be relaxed. Ben picks up a sandwich, examines the calories and fat content, and then puts it down again. Then another. And another. Suddenly he spies something advertised as a "half-fat" sandwich: half the fat because it's literally only half a sandwich.

"No, you're not having that," I whisper loudly, trying to ignore the curious glances from people pushing past us in the queue. Ben picks up another sandwich and puts it down, then picks up another and puts that down, too, then slams one - at random - onto the tray and propels himself and the sandwich towards the till. I breathe a sigh of relief and take my sandwich along, too.

As the cashier reaches for his food to scan it through the till, Ben suddenly does a U-turn. The sandwich ends up back on the shelf.

There's another attempt to get as far as the till. Another sandwich goes back on the shelf. Ben's face is reddening; I can sense the hysteria rising. My heart sinks. Suddenly he leaves his tray where it is and flees across the café, crouching beneath the staircase where he begins to sob noisily in full view of the other diners. I mean, *really* noisily and obviously, like he used to do when he was a baby. Not that I give a damn about the diners' shocked stares.

Moments later he flees from the café in terror and heads up the main shopping street. I run after him, trying to keep up as he weaves in and out of the crowds of Saturday shoppers: normal people looking normal, behaving normally and doing normal shopping in the normal world that's parallel to ours.

I grab Ben's arm and steer him towards the bagel café in the cinema complex. "We're eating here," I announce abruptly, propelling him inside. And, to my surprise, we do. We successfully order savoury and sweet bagels, and frozen yoghurt. Ben eats most of it, saying he feels "guilty" as he leaves half a sweet bagel. By now my stress levels are sky high, all thoughts of shopping gone from my mind. I just want to go home. I spend the rest of the day curled up in bed - one of my get-away-from-the-demon sanctuaries.

As I explain to Ben years later when he accuses me of over-reacting: "We'd just had the meltdown from hell in Pret. And it wasn't just that; it was the culmination of everything that was going on at that time, 24/7. Already you'd lost tons of weight, transformed beyond all recognition and been in hospital with a dangerously low heart rate." I tell him that, back then, I had no idea where it was leading or even if we'd ever come through it.

"The pressure was immense. I was exhausted. Sometimes I just had to take time out and retreat. Like on this particular day. Yes you did eat lunch after the Pret fiasco, and yes I was relieved, but I'd reached the end of my coping. I also knew that it would probably happen again. And again…"

THE DEMON STAYS AWAY until the evening meal on Day Three of *Eating Plan 6* when I make the mistake of giving Ben a larger than normal portion which confuses him.

The demon arrives with a vengeance screeching, "I'm fat!" at the top of Ben's voice, bashing Ben's head with Ben's fists. Ben is in meltdown again. "I hate myself! I hate, hate, hate myself!" He smashes a fist onto his plate, mushing up the food so it's inedible.

On Monday Ben accidentally-on-purpose misses the bus, so I insist on driving him to school. A text is waiting for me when I get home. "I feel fat and horrid," it says. I ignore it, cross my fingers and hope he eats a proper school lunch.

Tuesday isn't so bad. We have a meeting with Linda which helps to take the pressure off for a while. But the demon is never away for long and by the next day it's back, attracted by the half naan bread I'm trying to get Ben to eat with his curry. The prospect of "fatty" carbs-laden bread sends him into a spiral of panic which gets worse when he discovers we're having lamb kebabs the next day. "I can't cope!" His scream reaches fever pitch. "I'll be thinking about it all day! *Is that what you want?"* Yet again the demon is punishing me for "force-feeding" him.

"Look," I insist, "You're strong. You can do it. Just give yourself a good talking to". He responds by slapping his face violently with his fists, over and over again. Eventually, to my surprise, he sits down and eats the meal, saying he doesn't want to talk about it.

The following day I bottle out and allow the lamb kebabs to be swapped for a low fat chicken burger. But even that doesn't placate the demon. I can see it scanning the burger buns, relishes and toppings on the table.

"There's too much choice!" Ben yells. "I don't know where to start! I don't know what I should have. I can't tell if I'm having too much or too little. I just don't know!"

He begins to pick up stuff and put it down again, flitting from one dish to another. He crashes his fists down on the plate sending food flying. But, like yesterday, he eventually calms down and eats.

Unfortunately the demon isn't happy with the way Ben's calmed down and eaten his meal. Later that evening Ben suddenly throws down the book he's reading. Crash, bang! "I'm fat!" he howls, smashing his fists onto the coffee table and thumping the furniture. "I don't need all this food you're forcing me to eat. My old diet was fine!" Arguing with him is useless; I might as well be talking in Chinese. He keeps repeating the same irrational words over and over again. It's as if he hates me.

By the next day Ben has calmed down. I keep him off school and we spend most of the day on the sofa, talking. I put my arm around his shoulder, trying to get to the heart of the matter. Much of the time he just sits and sobs, or curls up in a ball while I talk quietly and, I hope, encouragingly.

I pray he's listening and hope it's going in. But his mind is busy whirring around like a machine, calculating calories and fat, working out how much exercising he'll need to do to burn off the food he's just eaten and worrying about what we'll be eating later. "I can't eat those scotch pancakes you bought, mum," he says out of the blue. "They're 85 calories each."

All he's been thinking about are scotch pancakes.

He hasn't been listening to a single word I've said.

The next evening Ben is sitting on the sofa when I'm suddenly aware of him looking down, eyes fixed on his belly. I know what's coming next. He lifts his sweater and pinches the "rolls of fat" and prods his "double chin". "Can't you see how fat I'm getting?" He squeezes the folds of skin viciously. "Can't you see you're making me fat! You, dad and CAMHS - you all want to make me fat!"

Arguing is pointless.

On Monday we have a meltdown over lunch. "I'm greedy!" he

screeches, "Can't you see I'm overeating?" and suddenly we're back to pinching the stomach folds and "waist fat". He slaps his palms against his "fat" belly. "Can't you see that I'm going to blob out if I go on like this?" He looks at me desperately, as if I've gone mad, as if I don't understand the most obvious fact in the universe.

"Everyone's ignoring me, I'm a social outcast, I f*cking hate myself. And they say I'm fat! No wonder they do when I'm not being allowed to exercise!" For the time being, Ben's banned from PE and games, but he's still exercising at home.

He insists I weigh him. I refuse. He's itching to get weighed and charges out of the room desperately trying to find where I've hidden the scales. Thankfully I've hidden them well.

Then Ben discovers we're having curry for supper again. "You're destroying my life! I don't need to eat all this food!" he shrieks. "Can't you see how fat I am? Other people can!"

"Who can?" I ask aghast. No reply. I could throttle whoever it was who shouted "Run, fat boy, run!" on one of his many runs to the park and back. *What are people on, for God's sake?* Or the Year 9 boy at school whose gang crowded round Ben, taking the mickey, as he hid at the top of a little-used staircase to eat his packed lunch.

These days Ben pinches his "fat gut" virtually every evening. It is agonising for us to watch him scrunch those loose folds of skin, pinching them until bruises begin to show. "Look! I'm fat!" he screams the next evening, prodding his belly viciously. He begins to pull out his hair in clumps. "Fat, fat, fat!" He gets up from the sofa, runs to the wall and bashes his skull against it, slapping his face with his fists, before charging upstairs and barricading himself in his room. I rush after him and push against the door, but it doesn't budge. He's holding it shut. He weighs less than I do - and I'm only small yet, uncannily, he's far stronger than me.

Eventually I force myself into the room. Ben grabs me by the shoulders and begins to shake me violently. "Where have you hidden the scales?" Again I refuse to tell him. "I'm going to find them!" He begins to pull clothes and books out of cupboards and wardrobes. But even the demon can't find where I've hidden the scales.

By Wednesday Ben is panicking about the size of his "fat gut". His entire happiness seems to centre round the perceived size of his belly which always leads to the need-to-exercise-it-off mind set. That evening he suddenly looks at his belly and prods it, yelling that he's fat, fat, fat… disgustingly fat. Then we're back to the head banging: the skull hammering that makes me grit my teeth as I wait for the sound of shattering bone. Good grief, the human skull must be strong. But, then, we've always joked that Ben's head is made from concrete.

LOOKING BACK ON our early CAMHS sessions, I have no memory of being shown how to implement *Eating Plan 6* successfully; I am just aware of "doing it" and making copious notes on Ben's daily reactions and behaviours. These notes, I assumed, would be used to discuss and analyse Ben's progress. In the event I don't remember my notes being used at all - except to help me put this book together.

Aside from the eating plan, I do remember being asked at one of the very first CAMHS sessions to write a letter about what I, as a parent, would say to the anorexia if it were a person. Again, I assumed we would be discussing this at a future session. It was never referred to again.

Evil Anorexia,

I can't address you as "Dear" because I loathe and hate you more than anything I've ever hated before in my life.

You are an evil little sneak that crept into our family, uninvited, even earlier than we thought you had. You saw our happy family. You saw my good looking, bright, sporty, friendly and confident son, in fact you probably homed in on him around the time I was feeling so mega proud that this young man… this handsome individual who girls would pass in the street, admire and turn round to take a second glance… this wonderful, amazing young man was MY gorgeous son. I made him! Incredible!

So you decided to ruin all this. You sneaked in and took over his mind, only you disguised it as normal behaviour for many months so we didn't realise you were there. Being with Ben every day we didn't notice the subtle changes, many of which were disguised as "normal" behaviour. It was only when Ben's grandma visited in September and commented on his appearance that we realised he had changed so much.

Actually, you know, I could write pages and pages about why I hate you so much. But I'm not going to do that. Instead, I'm going to tell you how we plan to send you packing, to expel you from inside Ben until not one ounce of your evil remains - and I will get my wonderful "little boy" back - before you eat up the rest of his remaining "childhood".

One thing you hadn't banked on was how strong Paul and I are. We're not the kind of parents who give up on things; we're fighters. And we will fight tooth and nail where our beloved son is concerned, the most precious possession we have in the world and our reason for living.

For me, this started when I gave birth. It was a horrible birth - but the bonding I made with Ben took me by surprise. I knew that, given poorer medical care, one or both of us could have died during the birth.

What I felt as we both lay there… me battered, bruised and cut… was a primeval instinct. It was almost animal in its intensity - a case of me and Ben against the world. I knew at that moment that I would love and protect Ben forever and give my life for him if needs be.

And I know Paul thinks the same.

If I were you, evil Anorexia, I'd slink off back to your nasty, dark, damp evil little hole. You don't stand a chance with us. Okay, it might involve some "tough love" on our part - but you know it's not Ben we'd be talking to, it's you. We've known Ben long enough to know who the "real Ben" is. A lot of what we are seeing now isn't him at all; it's you. The thing is, we know when it's you that's talking or lying - you can't get away from us now that we recognise you!

Okay, so there are little things you do because you think that if you've failed with one thing you'll get away with another. Your aim is to stop Ben from eating by hook or by crook - and also make him so depressed he runs to you for comfort. Well, your days are numbered, mark my words. We know who you are and we know what you sound like.

*We don't want you in our house any longer. We don't want you in our lives. We don't want you in our son. So sod off, you little sh*t, back to where you came from and leave us - and our son - alone and never come back.*

And don't think you can return at any point like when Ben's at university or whatever.

I'm not going to waste any more time writing to you.

Ben's Mum

Following our second CAMHS session after the production of *Eating Plan 6*, I note that Ben seems fairly normal. Until I mention that it's time for his snack. "Do I have a snack? Do I *need* a snack? *Should* I have a snack? I don't know if I should have a snack?" I can hear him getting hysterical. The anorexia has robbed him of the ability to make rational decisions.

On Friday I'm brave enough to take Ben into the city centre and attempt another lunch at Pret. My stress levels are stratospheric as I watch him dart from one sandwich to another, picking stuff up and putting it down, just like last time. I say nothing; I just stand there. What seems like an age later he makes a decision. Keep the sandwich on the tray… Phew! Wow! We make it past the till. And then he eats it, every bit, while I pretend it's just a normal day. Afterwards, to my surprise, he suggests we go to Starbucks for a skinny latte. Another success. Skinny latte is better than no latte.

But before I can steer him past the chocolate shop next door, he's inside like a shot, its mountains of temptingly wrapped chocolates attracting him like a magnet.

He spends the next 30 minutes or so examining the nutritional content of every single chocolate bar, picking stuff up, putting it down, admiring the creative displays, desperate to buy something. At one point he almost does.

Almost.

13

pear-shaped & messy

IT'S SATURDAY AFTERNOON and we've gone to the theatre to see Alan Bennett's *The History Boys.* Desperate for Ben to stick to the eating plan, I've brought the obligatory snack for him to have in the interval. Paul and I grab a coffee, but Ben disappears off somewhere.

I catch him in the theatre café, examining the large display cabinet, its glass shelves laden with gooey, creamy cakes. It's the café-in-the-park charade all over again. And again we have to send away the assistant when she comes over to take his order. How can I explain that Ben has no intention of eating any of this? Not now. Not ever. He manages to avoid having his snack, too, and the fruit juice I've brought along.

Ever the brave family, we stop off at Pizza Express on the way home in a parody of the happy family having a wonderful day out. To ensure everything runs smoothly I've done some prep, printing out the online menu with its nutritional information for Ben to take with him to keep him calm. Ben's even walked me through what he plans to order.

By now our stress levels are sky-high. Paul and I are on a knife-edge. One false move and - pow! - the whole show could implode. Ben orders a pizza. So far so good. Not a slimline pizza, either, but a standard pizza. Shame he's gone for the diet drink, though, and the fat-reduced mozzarella. As the meal progresses I'm aware of Ben getting quieter, pushing the pizza crust around the plate.

The waitress comes over to see if we've finished. "How was your meal?"

"It was lovely, thanks," Paul says.

"No it wasn't," Ben pipes up. "It was bland. I didn't enjoy it at all." I can see the tell-tale red flush spreading across his face.

Suddenly the demon is back, right there with us, in Pizza Express, in full view of all the Saturday evening diners. My heart does its usual thud as my body goes ice cold, terrified of what the demon has in store for us next.

Ben is creating a scene. A big scene. Everyone is pretending not to notice and it's embarrassing. I'm pretending not to care. The waitress rushes over again. "Everything's fine," we assure her with fake smiles as Ben noisily flees from the restaurant into the night. "Sorry about that," I say, avoiding the looks of the other diners. "It's just that..." My voice tails off. I can't even begin to explain why my teenage son is behaving like he is.

We find Ben some way down the main road standing on the kerb looking as if he's about to throw himself in front of the traffic. We plead with him to come home, but the demon is raging. I attempt to hug him, but he pushes me to the ground violently. Paul drags him off me. Screaming, Ben flies off down the road towards our house.

"I can't take any more of this!" Paul sobs. I mean, *really* sobs. Paul, a former rugby player, is sobbing like a baby. Our son has become a monster and we're powerless to do anything about it.

"I feel bloated and uncomfortable," Ben complains the next day when presented with a sandwich containing low fat spread. "I feel faint and can't stop sweating. And I've got cramps in my guts!" I tell him that he can't continue with sandwiches made from dry bread; he must add butter or spread.

Later Paul catches him pouring half a smoothie down the sink. At suppertime, he discreetly throws some of his yoghurt into the trash bin before eating the remainder in front of us, pretending that it's the whole pot. It's only later that Paul discovers the other half in the bin, concealed in a piece of kitchen paper. We begin to police the kitchen whenever Ben is in there with his food. He always seems to have some excuse about why he needs to go back into the kitchen. So we go back in there with him. And we observe him closely. He doesn't like it.

Ben continues to complain of stomach cramps at breakfast when I persuade him to finish the crumpets he's discarded after just two bites. "I don't need to eat all this stuff!" he yells, "My weight is okay as it is!"

Then at lunchtime he texts me from school to protest about the calories in his sandwich: "It's far too much! I don't need it!" The eating-too-much argument continues at suppertime and way into the evening including an absurd fight about the horrors of low fat yoghurts versus fat-free ones.

Reasoning with your anorexic child is pointless. My son who is an A-star student and whose encyclopaedic mind is crammed full of facts and figures about history, politics, philosophy, evolution and a host of other complex topics - and who is always the first to correct anyone if they get a fact wrong - is doing the equivalent of insisting that the world is flat when everyone knows it's round.

The following day he freaks out at the thought that he might have to eat high calorie food in the future - food like butter or ordinary yoghurt. "I have no idea if CAMHS will insist you do or not," I say. "They might want to ease it in or they might not. I don't know, I can't say."

I have begun to act like the poor ignorant little mother just doing what the professionals tell her to do. In other words, I'm doing a very good job of sitting on the fence. Let the demon take it out on CAMHS for a change. I'm sick to the back teeth of getting the blame.

"I will *never* eat this stuff! *Ever!*" I can hear the hysteria rising in his voice. "And CAMHS don't listen to me when I explain *why* I will *never* eat this stuff, *ever!*"

Ben arrives back from school the next day complaining of heartburn and bloating. "It's just how I used to feel when I was fat! That's why I started to lose weight in the first place!" he shrieks. "Can't you see? I'm getting fat again, just like I was then!" He sobs on my shoulder begging me to give up the eating plan and to ask CAMHS to focus on "getting my head sorted out". He looks at me with puppy-like pleading eyes. "I feel so boated and flabby, mum. And, you know, I really shouldn't be eating this much - I really shouldn't." He's like a little boy all over again. "Mum," he implores, "You do realise I'm eating *double* what a normal boy eats?" But I stand my ground and we end up having the usual vicious circle arguments before he rushes up to his room, coming down a short while later, coughing and eyes streaming, announcing that the cramps have made him vomit.

On Monday morning, Ben tries to leave his lunchbox in the car after a massive row on the way to the school bus stop. He's been throwing toast around the kitchen, shouting that he doesn't want to do the eating plan any longer. "CAMHS just want to make me fat!" he screams. He spends most of the day in the school medical centre with Sheila, the nurse. At lunchtime he texts me with "The eating plan is making me lonelier than ever. I can't talk to people any more…"

Still no-one has shown me how to implement the "proper" *Eating Plan 6*. In fact no-one has shown me how to do anything, really, because many of the CAMHS sessions have been individual sessions between Ben and Sarah while I sit in the waiting room. We've seen Alice, the dietician, a couple of times and she's doing her best to push the benefits of fats and help Ben to overcome his long list of fear foods. But Ben's not listening. Or he's distorting her words into his own twisted version of "healthy eating". Fat is still Public Enemy Number One. So, for the time being, we're stuck with the tweaked version of the eating plan: the fat-free, carbs-high eating plan that fills Ben up until he feels as if he's going to explode. I'm not surprised he freaks out at the sheer quantity of food on his plate, accusing me of giving him an unbalanced meal and yelling at me for "going against Alice's advice". *But how the heck can I give him a balanced meal if he refuses to eat one?* The only alternative is to go back to the stuff he was eating before we began treatment - the diet that resulted in him losing a quarter of his bodyweight. So until we can devise a way of getting all those high calorie, low bulk foods into Ben, I'm afraid it's huge portions - or nothing.

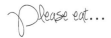

Of course none of this is helped by the fact that, before the anorexia, the three of us made a conscious decision to eat "healthily". Like many families, I suspect, we felt we were being good to our bodies by purchasing the kind of "healthy" products that, these days, fill me with alarm: low fat spread, skimmed milk, zero fat yoghurt, light mayonnaise... We viewed butter, cream and so on as the baddies; too much of that sort of thing and your arteries would fur up faster than you could say cardiac arrest. We grilled rather than fried, and never deep-fried anything. We opted for olive or rapeseed oil rather than vegetable oil, butter, lard or the arch baddie of them all: hydrogenated fat. I kick myself as I remember the days when I'd stand at the supermarket checkout with my "lite" this and "zero fat" that feeling oh so self-righteous as the woman in front of me packed pizzas, pies, cream cakes and puddings into her bags. Look at us; we are so H-E-A-L-T-H-Y, I wanted to brag.

So suddenly doing a U-turn and extolling the virtues of doughnuts, cream and all-butter pastry feels hypocritical - like preaching the gospel when everyone knows you're a hardened atheist. I'm not surprised that Ben's accusing me of being two-faced. "Why would I suddenly eat this kind of thing when we've *never* eaten it?" he yells at me.

"But you're not on a diet, Ben!" I scream for the hundredth time.

Yet again I'm faced with the frustration of having access to all the food Ben needs yet he refuses to eat anything other than diet options.

TO HIS CREDIT BEN MANAGES to stick to my tweaked version of *Eating Plan 6* for a few more weeks. Yes, we fight like cat and dog about it. Yes, his diet it still low in fats and high in bulk. And, yes, he takes so long to eat that one meal runs into another, but we succeed. So much so that the scales soon begin to register a steady weight gain which, of course, reinforces his belief that he doesn't need fats in his diet. I can rattle off all the science until I'm blue in the face, but he just yells at me: "I already get enough fat! I eat the same amount of fat as an obese person!!!"

I try another tactic. "I eat loads more fat than you... butter, cheese, pastry, chocolate... and it hasn't made me obese!" And I'm only 5ft 3, middle aged, female... *Will someone fix that stuck record?*

I get lectured at, like a sergeant major scolding errant troops. I get the full distorted healthy eating lecture about the horrors of fats, especially saturated fat, and the shocking things that overconsumption of fat can do to the human body.

I get constantly reminded of those TV programmes we used to watch where I'd recoil in horror at the frightening amount of fat people were consuming before following the TV doctor's sensible diet plan. Trying to get Ben to eat fats is becoming an impossible task. I feel as if I'm trying to persuade him to take strychnine.

It's something that never fails to astonish me. The way people with eating disorders can insist they're eating an ultra-healthy diet when, in fact, they're doing untold damage to their bodies: bones, internal organs and muscle... The thing is, ever since he took up sport, Ben's been interested in eating and drinking healthily. He knows the science back to front. He knows the facts. Yet, since the anorexia took hold, he's distorted this into something that's blatantly untrue. Dangerously untrue. I just don't get it.

Meanwhile CAMHS are delighted that Ben has put on weight. To be truthful, he doesn't look too bad... quite skinny, yes... but not too bad. If you didn't know he had an eating disorder, or hadn't seen him back in the rugby playing days, you might think he was naturally thin. And at CAMHS Ben is all sweetness and light. He's the model patient, apparently cooperating with the eating plan, agreeing to do the cognitive homework Sarah sets for him and - most importantly - putting on weight.

Yet I know he's still very sick. The trouble is I'm not convinced that CAMHS agree with me. I really believe they think *I'm* the one with the problem, not Ben. I am too anxious. I worry too much. And of course the demon has taken their side. Big Bad Mum versus Kind Caring CAMHS.

I wish Sarah and Linda could visit our home and experience what it's like to see your once beautiful, confident and popular child disintegrate into a crumpled wreck of a human being, just because he's spotted the calorie content of the bread we're having with our evening meal.

I wish they could see him collapsing on the floor into a quivering mess of sobbing, banging his head against the wall as if he's about to break his skull.

I wish they could see him striding around the house trying to find where I've hidden the scales. Or shake me with such force that his dad has to physically prise him off me.

But they don't see any of this.

All they see is a model patient who is cooperating with the eating plan and whose BMI is already creeping into what the charts consider to be a healthy range.

The demon is revelling in the charade.

Meanwhile I'm still unclear about what kind of treatment Ben is receiving for his eating disorder other just talking things over with Sarah. At the end of April I send a note to CAMHS asking what their plans are for "the immediate and distant future". Paul and I want to see some kind of tangible "game plan" together with idea of "how the treatment will take place and what it will be", especially as - by this time - Ben is only seeing CAMHS once every two weeks. I also ask for a "proper personalised eating plan".

"When will Ben's treatment begin?" I remember asking CAMHS at one point.

"This is it!" they said. "It's already begun!"

But to me, feeling helpless and hopeless, it seems like the Emperor's New Clothes. I'm supposed to be seeing something, but in reality I can't see anything at all.

Except Ben disappearing off a precipice.

14
school's out

EVERY DAY BEN TEXTS me from school: frantic texts about how fat he's feeling or worries about what I'm planning for the evening meal.

One day it pushes me over the edge. I've asked Sheila if Ben can eat his packed lunch with her in the medical centre. This way she can check that he eats it and, hopefully, it's not as stressful as eating with everyone else in the canteen. Today Ben is supposed to be eating a chicken sandwich. But Sheila's been called out on an emergency and so he's in the medical centre alone.

"I can't eat the sandwich and have a burger tonight," says the first text. "I can't do it!" says the second followed by "No! There's way too much and the chicken's really fatty" in response to my replies of "Eat it".

A deluge of texts follows.

"It's too much!" "I can't stand this!" "I hate this feeling!" "What am I gonna do? I've had my snack things and pud yet I haven't had quite enough yet it's too late to have anything and yet I'm having a big supper tonight so really I have had enough." "That friggin' sandwich has ruined my day more than it was already!" "F*ck it! I can't stand this! Too confusing! Have I had enough? Have I done enough? Should I go home? Am I doing enough for it? Is supper too big? Was my lunch too big? Why am I doing nothing? Is it too late to eat? Was what I had for lunch actually the right amount? Should I eat more? Why do people distance me? Will I ever be normal?!"

Text after text after text, like a horrific avalanche. Higher and higher my stress levels go until they can go no higher. I pick up a pile of dinner plates that has been sitting on the kitchen work surface and smash them onto the tiled floor. Then I grab some more. Smash! Smash, smash, smash! More, more, more! What else can I break? Smish, smash, smish!

I crumple into a ball in the corner of the kitchen surrounded by yellow and blue shards of crockery. This time it's me that's wailing like a wounded animal, rocking to and fro. Thoughts whiz around my head like a hellish game of pinball. All those hopes and dreams I had for Ben… the hopes and dreams he had for himself… smashed to smithereens by this hellish illness. All that love I've invested, all those hours and hours talking, of pleading, of trying to understand, of trying to find solutions, of desperately trying to make him well…

I realise with horror that I no longer recognise my child. My darling son, my beautiful handsome boy who was thriving in every way… so talented… so popular… My boy has completely vanished and I don't know if I'll ever get him back.

Hot tears stream down my face. I grab a nearby tea-towel and wipe it across my eyes, blowing my nose noisily. I've given everything… everything I could possibly give I've given. All those sleepless nights… all that praying… all that standing there and taking it while the anorexia demon hurls abuse at me or threatens to destroy my dear child.

I just don't have the strength to fight this anymore… I am empty. *I am just a mum…* a mum who loves her child and wants him back. Whole. Happy. Alive. That's all I want. Nothing more. "Is this too much to ask?" I plead with the empty kitchen as if it can help me. "I've done everything I can." I feel as if I've failed.

I sink deeper onto the floor, wrapping my arms around my wet, aching head. But I know there is no-one around to comfort me, no-one to tell me it's going to be okay and no-one to support or care for me - the parent who is going through this nightmare. I feel so utterly helpless and alone. My head thumps with pain. I crawl upstairs to my bed and just lie there, refusing to take any more texts or messages. Let the school deal with him. I'm completely spent. I can't function. I cry until my tears dry up. And then I cry until they're dry again. I feel totally, utterly broken, sapped by the leechlike ability of Ben's anorexia to suck me dry of every last ounce of my being until all that's left is an empty shell.

I am just so dog tired. Dog, dog, dog tired. My teeth, my brain, my skull and my cheeks ache. I wish I could just sleep. I wish I could just fall into a deep, blissful sleep and never wake up… I don't know what a blissful sleep is any more.

"What if this is the pattern for the rest of our lives?" I shout out to the empty bedroom. "I couldn't do it. *I just couldn't do it.*"

How I long for someone to take care of me. Someone to swoop in, take charge, sweep me up in their arms and look after me. More than anything, I just want someone to give me a great big physical hug.

When Paul comes home from work I show him the bags of broken crockery waiting to be taken to the bin. "Well that didn't really achieve anything, did it?" is his insensitive response. Not the sympathetic reply I'd hoped for, and definitely not the great big hug I so desperately need. I feel like doing it all over again.

That night, after a scene over the bread roll that Ben was supposed to be having with the burger, I reach the end of my coping. I tell Paul we must remove Ben from school while we focus on recovery full time. Yes he has his GCSE exams in a couple of months - Ben is an A-star pupil and expected to excel - but, hey, what can we do; recovery comes first.

The next day I make an appointment with the Headmaster to talk about Ben and school. These days we can't leave Ben in the house alone, not for a moment. I get my mum to sit with him while Paul and I go into school.

We arrive in the car park at 8.30am just before the bell goes. Scores of boys and girls are heading towards the main school, laughing, joking and looking impossibly healthy. We are both thinking the same: *This should be Ben.*

We are ushered into the Headmaster's office. The Head of Year is called into the meeting too. "First let me say that, as a fellow parent, I can't imagine what you are going through," says the Head sympathetically. He says that whatever the school can do to help they will attempt to do it.

I explain that Ben is finding it too stressful to be in school. By now he can scarcely bear to be with his peers for five minutes let alone a full school day. I point out that he's hardly in lessons these days; he just goes to pieces and usually ends up hiding in a corner somewhere. I tell him we'd like to remove Ben from school temporarily. This way we can focus on his recovery full time. But I also stress that Ben needs intellectual stimulation; it takes his mind off the eating disorder.

"What if we arrange for Ben's tutors to send work home for him, via email, and where email isn't possible then you can come into school - say, once a week - to drop off work to be marked? I can't see there being a problem; we've made similar arrangements for other pupils in the past and it's worked well."

It sounds perfect.

"But what about the GCSE exams?" I ask. We are worried that if Ben suddenly finds himself amongst his peers he might freak out making it impossible for him to do the exams. And make it impossible for the others to do theirs, too.

"I am sure we can arrange for him to sit his exams separately." The Headmaster goes on to emphasise that the school will do whatever it takes to make things as easy as possible for Ben. "I'm sure we can set up a Plan A, Plan B, even a Plan C if necessary."

I am so relieved I could dance. Or, at least, I would if I wasn't so shattered. I am so very, very tired that I could sleep forever.

But, thankfully, the Headmaster's plan works. Studying at home reduces Ben's anxiety and keeps him stimulated. Having him at home also means I can monitor him closely and be certain that he eats his meals. Just as important, he and I can talk.

We quickly fall into a daily routine. Ben studies in the morning and in the afternoon we go for a walk - or we just talk at home, go shopping or visit a museum or gallery. Without the pressure of school and school dinners, Ben brightens up a little and I manage to catch a few nights' unbroken sleep.

IT'S MOTHERS' DAY, the day when all mothers across the country are spoiled rotten. Breakfast in bed, children offering to do the chores, maybe an outing, a special lunch or dinner... At our house the demon gate crashes the day.

Following some disagreement over a snack the demon explodes into a magnificent rage. On this day of all days he rants, screams and swears. By the afternoon I've had enough. I pick up a box of tissues, the box of chocolates Ben has given me and my car keys, and get into the car. Unable to think straight, I drive this way and that - first north, then south, then north again - out into the countryside and up onto the moorland. I sit on a hillside for some time, overlooking fields of sheep, sobbing into the tissues and eating the chocolates mechanically one after the other, my heart broken.

In the evening we manage to go out to a local country pub for a Mothers' Day meal. But you can almost physically feel the stress as Ben's meal is placed on the table in front of him: salmon and new potatoes, glistening with melted butter. I eye the yellow liquid with terror praying that he won't notice it. Thankfully he eats everything and, to my surprise, goes on to order - and eat - a sticky toffee pudding and ice cream. But the meal ends with Ben fleeing to the gents' toilets mortified at what he's just consumed. Paul follows him swiftly; somehow we both know that Ben will be doing some kind of exercise in an attempt to wear off the meal. Probably punching the air or doing star jumps.

"The anorexia didn't want me to eat," Ben would say a couple of years later. "But I did. I ate every bit. It was my way of trying to make amends for earlier in the day."

That night I have a horrible nightmare. I wake up sweating, my heart beating fast. In it we've been given a new psychiatrist of the "old school" variety - really scary and strict. This psychiatrist is telling me off and shouting at me that I should be feeding Ben far more than I am doing, especially fats. I end up yelling at her, "How the heck do you expect me to get the food into him when he refuses to eat!" Ben is promptly taken away by "the men in white coats" to a prison-like institution. Staff refuse to let me near him as I try desperately to give him a hug.

In my daydreams I imagine a kind of large, motherly nanny character - like the "super nanny" on the TV programme - who arrives on our doorstep and takes charge. She feeds Ben (successfully), calms him down (successfully) and cares for him (successfully). She refuses to take any nonsense. She is in total control. Me, well I just sit back, breathe out slowly and let her get on with it.

Actually, Linda tells me one day, there's a team that will come into your house at meal times to help your child eat. Or at least she thinks it's in the process of being set up. My heart leaps. But I hear nothing more about it.

OVER THE NEXT MONTH or so Ben's weight gradually goes up. One day the scales show a very slight increase which just tips him into what the charts consider to be a "healthy" BMI.

"Congratulations!" say CAMHS, all smiles. "You've just scraped into the healthy weight range!" Of course Ben takes this to mean that he is fully weight restored and doesn't need to put on any more

So, when I continue to enforce the eating plan, he panics at the prospect of ballooning out into a "huge, fat, flabby monster". He makes the decision to cut back. That night he sits on the sofa pinching the "rolls of fat" on his belly to "prove" he's right.

Later I switch on my laptop, click on My Pictures and scroll down to the summer of 2008 - the summer that Ben did the Coast2Coast cycle ride and we went on holiday to the south of France.

There's a photo of Paul and Ben striding out of the sea. Ben's broad shoulders are pink with too much sun, and his torso, arms and legs are "rippling" with muscle.

Yes, the charts may be showing that Ben has just crept into what is considered to be a "healthy" BMI range, but the boy I'm looking at now is a faint shadow of the broad-shouldered strapping young man striding out of the sea.

ONE DAY AT LUNCHTIME Ben says he isn't "hungry". He refuses to eat the egg which he was going to have: "Too hard boiled." The date and walnut cake I've made is "too dry", so I suggest having ice cream instead but he's "just not hungry".

I insist he eats something and calmly explain the reasons why he needs to eat. "I'll get you some ice cream," I say in a fake calm voice.

"Okay, if you want me to have ice cream, I'll have f*cking ice cream!" The demon is screaming in that deeper-than-deep, sinister voice which is so very different from Ben's real voice. The voice that makes my blood freeze. Dragging open the freezer compartment drawer, he pulls out the ice cream tub and proceeds to shovel ice cream into his mouth. Spoon after spoon goes in before he spits the contents of his mouth onto the floor.

I look at him as calmly as I can. "When I come back I want to see this mess cleaned up." I head for my sanctuary at the bottom of the garden. Every step towards the vegetable plot takes me further away from the demon and whatever it's doing to Ben in the house. It's one of the "safe places" I go to when I can't take any more.

A few days later, following a snack, I find a chewed up cereal bar in the toilet. Ben insists that it was stuck in his throat and that's why he spat it out.

It's getting harder and harder to implement the eating plan. God only knows how he would have coped with the real *Eating Plan 6* not this low calorie, minimal fat hybrid. Now Ben's weight has crept into the "healthy" range, it looks less and less likely that we'll ever follow the real plan. As Ben keeps insisting over and over again, "I've got into the safe BMI range without the need to eat fat". So why the heck would he start to eat it now?

I feel as if the dietician has got her work cut out.

Getting Ben to eat fats is like getting him to take poison.

15

master of deception

THE TROUBLE WITH ANOREXIA is that many people just don't "get it". As a result you can feel terribly alone, as if you're living in a parallel world to everyone else.

The good news is, though, that Ben's anorexia has meant that we've discovered who our real friends are: those wonderful, selfless, loving and supportive people who don't just care about what's happening to our family but who are willing to go through a massive learning curve in an attempt to understand it.

Along the line other friends have moved off the radar; friends who avoid us for whatever reason. Maybe they can't understand or they just don't want to understand. Or perhaps it's because they have their own problems to deal with. Also, anorexia has become such a huge part of my life that I find it difficult to talk about anything else. I have become an "anorexia bore".

When anorexia dominates your every waking moment it's virtually impossible to make any social plans. I never know from one day to the next where Ben's mood will take us (usually to hell and back…) And - to be frank - when I'm in floods of tears most of the time, I'm not very good company.

But some people are more than willing to be in on our "secret", whatever the cost, and it's around this time that I meet Sue.

One Sunday morning I'm desperate to find a willing ear - someone that will be there for me, who won't mind me ranting on about the eating disorder. Certainly I have my wonderful sister and mum who are highly supportive, but I don't want to over-burden them. I decide to give the local church a try.

I walk into the building on my own, nervous and anxious, and sit on the back row. A few people stare in my direction, but no-one talks to me. I sit there feeling awkward and out of place, my emotions on a roller coaster.

I glance over my shoulder at the exit. The door is still wide open. Just a couple of strides and I could be out of the building and back to my car in minutes. The pull is magnetic.

I'm about to leave when - out of the corner of my eye - I'm aware of a tiny woman walking quickly towards me down the aisle, a huge smile on her face. She introduces herself as Sue and invites me to sit with her. Over the next 24 months, Sue will become my best and most supportive friend.

I think the main reason Sue gets it is because of the cancer: secondary breast cancer that's spread to her bones, liver and lungs. Over coffee after the service we sidestep the small talk and get straight to the heart of the matter. Within minutes I feel as if I've known Sue for ever. I know all about her cancer and she knows all about the anorexia. No chit-chat, no trivia, no small talk. Sue has well and truly taken me under her wing.

The thing about Sue is that, no matter how bad her own prognosis, she is always cheerful and smiling, and positive about the future. She also has a knack of turning the focus onto me and my problems, eager to learn all about Ben and his illness. She doesn't stop until she knows and understands everything.

"Please don't ever think that your stress is any less than mine," she says when I tell her off for focusing on my problems instead of hers. "My problems are different. And, to be honest, it helps to talk about something other than cancer."

I spend many an hour in Sue's sitting room while she plies me with coffee and cake. No matter what the problem or what time of day or night, she makes sure I know that she is there for me. Sue is an angel in the truest sense.

Help comes from another quarter in spring 2010 when I stumble across an online forum called Around the Dinner Table and its parent website FEAST (Families Empowered and Supporting Treatment of Eating Disorders). The ATDT forum offers advice and support for parents of young people with eating disorders. It has members, moderators and mentors from every English speaking country in the world. From the very first moment I discover it, I know I've struck gold.

At last I'm amongst other parents who are going through the same kind of nightmare. Many have already come through it and I read their success stories over and over again. It quickly becomes clear that this is no ordinary internet forum. Sure, we all have our own online nicknames, but - before long - we are making friends on Facebook under our real names. We email, Skype, talk on the phone and - wherever possible - meet up in person, compare notes and offer each other mutual support. ATDT and the friends I make through it will become a lifeline for me.

ONE LUNCHTIME I MAKE BEN a sandwich from some leftover roast beef. Bad mistake. The beef is "dripping in fat". This is followed by one of those pointless going-round-in-circles-and-getting-nowhere arguments as I try to reason with the irrational demon.

"When we get to CAMHS on Friday and I've put on loads of weight because of your extreme diet plan, it'll all be your fault!" he screeches. "I'm going to make sure CAMHS know how much you're mistreating me and trying to fatten me up. They'll be horrified - especially now my weight is healthy. I just don't need all this stuff!"

"Fine, okay, you tell them, see if I care," I respond. I'm in one of those at-the-end-of-my-tether moods.

He charges upstairs and slams his bedroom door while I head off to the sanctuary of my vegetable patch to watch the potatoes growing. I dream of large jacket potatoes stuffed with bacon, butter and cheese served with a side of BBQ beans and coleslaw (made with high fat mayo, naturally, none of that confounded "extra-lite" stuff).

Later Ben comes downstairs and sits beside me, head on my shoulder and silent. It's his way of letting me know that the rages aren't him, they're the demon and he is sorry for upsetting me. These incidents are like the eye of the storm, an oasis of calm where we can attempt to get our heads back into gear, ready for the next onslaught.

ON THE SOCIAL FRONT we chalk up a success. Or at least that's how it appears on the surface. Ben's booked himself onto a history conference in a nearby city. His schoolmates are going, too. I drop him off mid-morning. It's pouring with rain so I decide to go shopping at the designer outlet on the other side of the city. The only trouble is everyone else seems to have had the same idea. I can't find a parking space, so I end up back at the school where the conference is being held. It's not worth driving the 20 miles back home, so I sit and wait for it to finish.

Although it's Saturday there are plenty of people around. A rugby match is just ending and the opposition's transport is waiting to take them home. I remember Ben playing rugby here once. I watch the boys as they head for the changing rooms, the rain making muddy streaks down their arms and legs. Once they're showered and changed, I expect they'll head for the canteen for a slap-up lunch before they go home. Probably burgers, beans and chips followed by pudding and custard. Ah, I remember those Saturday rugby lunches well: Ben and the other boys tucking in enthusiastically while the parents snacked on a sandwich lunch in the school hall.

Home matches were best. Ben's school laid on a splendid spread for the parents. Mrs F's homemade cookies and cakes were legendary, as were her scones and sandwiches. You could rely on the rugby boys to hoover up anything that was left over when they joined their parents in the school hall, showered, squeaky-clean and well fed, dressed in their smart school uniforms, dragging holdalls of evil smelling rugby kits behind them.

I remember the compost-like smell of muddy rugby kit. Back home, I'd attempt to clean off some of the dirt under the outside tap before rinsing thoroughly and throwing into the washing machine. Ben could sort out his rugby boots; I refused to touch those. Good grief, whoever thought that white rugby shorts were a good idea?

Suddenly I'm jolted back to the present by the sound of a text coming in on my mobile phone. I freeze; that's the standard reaction these days. Especially when I see it's from Ben. But it's only to ask me to drive round to the front of the building to pick him up.

Outside the ancient hall with its leaded windows and fancy Tudor brickwork, I'm delighted to see Ben hugging everyone goodbye, just like any normal teenager. Driving back home the talk is all positive. Ben is making plans. He'll contact so-and-so – and yes he gets on quite well with some of the kids in the year below, so maybe he'll go round with them at school. Indeed it looks as if a return to school is on the cards.

But of course the anorexia demon lies and deceives. It lulls you into a false sense of security. It has you completely fooled while it continues to do its dirty work.

One night - shortly after the conference - Ben has a total and utter meltdown. He goes to pieces and becomes a sobbing, emotional wreck. He's been subdued all day and I can tell something is wrong. All hell breaks loose during the evening meal.

"Stop it!" I shout as I chase him into the living room where he begins to viciously hammer his skull against the wall. "It's the anorexia doing this, not you - not the real Ben."

"No, mum, can't you see?" he howls, thumping his fists against the radiator as he crumples to the ground in a quivering heap of hot tears. "It's *not* the anorexia. This is the *Real Ben;* the *Real Me* that you're seeing. The calm, cooperative Ben that you sometimes see is the anorexia *pretending* to be me! This… this wreck that you see here… *this is the Real Me!"* I've never seen him like this before. It's as if his body and spirit have been completely broken and what is left is a brittle empty shell. He pulls his body into the foetal position on the floor, sobbing wildly.

Through the gulps and tears, the Real Ben confesses that he's been lying and play acting. He's been pulling the wool over CAMHS' eyes so they believe they're seeing progress. "You see, mum, that isn't me; it's the anorexia. *It is pure acting.* It isn't me!"

He confesses that he's been cheating on portion sizes and doing secret exercising. Lots of exercising. "All I think about is food and exercise, morning, noon and night. I can't think of anything else. The hours in between meals are just blanks to fill in until the next meal."

"But what about our walks in the countryside?"

"I only do that to burn calories!" he shrieks, the hysteria rising. "You think we're having a nice jolly time, walking and talking, but that's not me either, it's the anorexia. It's kidding you, mum, it's kidding everyone! Remember the history conference? I kept having to go to the toilets and exercise; I had no choice. Don't you see? While the others were having coffee or finishing their lunch, I was punching the air in the gents' and frantically running on the spot!"

I need to tell CAMHS urgently. But we're not seeing them for another two weeks. Meanwhile I'm battling to keep Ben on the straight and narrow while he resists the eating plan and threatens to "tell on me" to Sarah and Linda. The demon is stronger than ever, despite the Real Ben's desperate confession.

I begin to wonder how a 60-minute treatment session every week or fortnight will rid Ben of this terrifying illness. When, for God's sake, does the change take place? *How* does it take place? Do CAMHS just talk and talk to him until - like magic - it suddenly begins to make sense? Some days - in fact most days - I fear that the anorexia is here to stay. I have visions of Ben ending up like those young people that are still sick, well into their late twenties and beyond...

This is reinforced by the fact that Ben has begun to rebel against what's left of the tweaked eating plan. He's also body checking more than ever, refusing to eat any fats of any sort and constantly arguing with Paul and me - the old irrational arguments that are a complete waste of time.

I feel as if everything we've achieved has been given a "real kicking" as the eating disorder tries to get control again and suck Ben down - deep, deep down into the abyss until he's too far gone to climb back out again.

BUT, DESPITE THIS, THERE IS the odd chink of sunlight. One morning Ben surprises me by eating a peanut butter covered cinnamon and raisin bagel for breakfast. Then he goes into town and buys himself a mid-morning snack and a lunch, even offering to send me photographs to prove it. (His idea, not mine...) Finally, he arrives home with a chocolate bar. He's also come back armed with gifts he's bought with his pocket money "to say thank you for putting up with me through all of this".

I wipe a tear from my eye and give my far-too-thin but still beautiful son a great big bear hug. "You know what?" I say. "The best gift of all will be when you're completely recovered and we get our 'little boy' back."

We continue to hug each other, tears streaming down our faces.

16

big bad mum

AT THE NEXT CAMHS SESSION the demon is back. I want to have a quiet word with Sarah about the play acting. But she spirits Ben away so quickly I don't get the chance. And, as they have their 60-minute session, I know the demon won't mention it. Instead it spends the whole session convincing Sarah that what remains of "mum's eating plan" isn't doing him any favours.

Back home the demon is in its element. Ben refuses to eat anything that isn't a diet or zero fat food and continues to fly off the handle at meal times, screaming, shouting and head-banging, and brow-beating me into switching evening meal plans at the 11th hour for a safer recipe. Despite the Real Ben's recent confession, nothing has changed on the behaviour or eating front. I feel as if I've been rendered powerless while I just sit there and watch him eat what he likes - calorie counting still, yes, but deciding on his own daily limit. I'm far from happy, but there's little I can do.

The idea, from what I gather from a hurried five minutes I managed to grab with Sarah after the last session, is to experiment to see what the scales say in relation to how much Ben has eaten. Hopefully this will prove to him that he *does* need to eat more and won't suddenly balloon out into obesity. At the same time Alice and Sarah will continue to drip-feed the concept of introducing fats in order to make Ben's diet more balanced. And now that he's slipped into the healthy weight range, he's in a far safer place. In other words, he's not going to drop down dead tomorrow.

My natural instinct as a mother is to continue feeding him with the eating plan at the same time as working on the fats phobia and everything else. I'm impatient; I just want the "old" Ben back as quickly as possible. But Ben's already shown signs of cracking and rebelling, and Sarah believes a softly-softly approach is much more likely to work. Paul backs the decision saying "They're the professionals, you're just a mum. What do you know?"

Away from CAMHS the demon continues to rage and make my life unbearable. Often I'm terrified Ben will go too far and take his own life, either by accident or by design. It's as if he's been completely consumed. He is inconsolable.

"I want you to know you can call me whatever time of day or night," says Sue the next day. "Please don't hesitate, not for a moment. Just call me. If I can't come round, I'll send Dave round. We are here if you need us."

Sometimes my mum sits with Ben while I visit Sue which I try to do at least once a week. Much of the time I daren't leave him in the house alone. My sister, too, continues to be incredibly supportive. Often on Sundays, when Paul's at home to keep an eye on Ben, I rush over to her house sobbing as she hands me tissues, coffee and sympathy.

During the week, with Paul working away from Monday to Friday, the demon is making my life hell. It will devise all manner of emotional blackmail threats to stop me from phoning Paul for help, calling in Sue or Dave, or my sister and her partner - usually along the lines of Ben taking his own life or leaving home.

It's a difficult juggling act. In a bid to avoid the nightly rages, I find myself warning Ben in advance of meal plans and listing the ingredients I'll be using. God forbid if I sneak in any oil or other fear foods. Yet occasionally he'll surprise me by eating something challenging like chocolate. But what I'm not aware of is the sheer amount of punishing exercise he does afterwards to compensate.

For a while Ben's weight only decreases slightly and CAMHS are pleased with his overall progress. Meanwhile I'm finding it harder than ever to be Ben's carer at home because, whatever I say or do, the demon bites my head off: "CAMHS say you've got to take a back seat," it yells at me. "They say you're a naturally anxious person and you worry too much. It's not helpful to me!"

I urgently need to set up a private meeting with Sarah. I tell her about Ben's breakdown, about how the so-called improvements we've been seeing are false and that Ben is just play acting. I say that anorexia thoughts are controlling him more than ever. They control everything he does. He is completely trapped by them.

But Sarah is adamant that the softly-softly approach is the best one. Okay, part of me says I need to relax a bit and not be so paranoid that he'll take off into the depths of anorexia at the slightest reduction in calories. However the other part is desperate to get my son back and the sheer snail-like pace of the treatment is driving me to distraction. But - as I remind myself - no-one ever said it would be quick. Am I being too impatient? Am I worrying unduly? Are Ben's occasional trips into the land of the normal the chink of light at the end of the tunnel? Am I hindering progress by nagging and over-focusing on food?

I really don't know.

I haven't got a clue.

THE ROAD GETS ROCKY when Ben has to go into school on two consecutive days to sit his GCSE art exams in May. Each exam lasts several hours. Although the school has arranged for Ben to sit the exams alone in an ante-room, just outside the main art room, his stress levels begin to soar as the Big Day approaches.

The demon surfaces in all its horrific glory as Ben is faced with two problems: school and what he refers to as "sitting around all day doing nothing". In other words, unable to shoot off and do hundreds of sit-ups and press-ups or run round the school grounds. On the Sunday before the exams I rush over to my sister's for some TLC.

On Day One, Ben howls and swears all the way to school. By the time we arrive, he's in pieces. He can't even get out of the car. In the end he summons up enough courage to rush across the car park and through the other buildings to the art block, eyes firmly on the ground in case he bumps into anyone he knows. He spends the remainder of the two days trying to stay invisible.

He later confesses to me that - whenever the exam invigilator was out of the room - he immediately downed tools, lay on the floor and forced himself to do sit-ups, press-ups and crunches. Not surprisingly Ben doesn't get a great mark in GCSE art; Ben who is a natural at the subject and who is easily an A-star student.

On the plus side, Ben manages to go into school for the pre-exams English party. On the minus side, he flees from the classroom part-way through, unable to cope with all the canapés and cakes being served. Staff spend the best part of the morning trying to locate him. Eventually someone finds him curled up in a foetal position behind the school chapel, weeping. I get a call from the Deputy Head. Can I come in and take Ben home?

However Ben surprises me by successfully attending the Year 11 end-of-exams formal meal. Astonishingly, considering the recent school chapel incident, I have a handful of photos showing Ben messing around with his friends afterwards, looking much like any other boy, holding a pen in his teeth at a careless angle, his white school shirt covered in scrawled messages of goodwill. *Is this a chink of light at the end of the tunnel, I wonder?*

Back at CAMHS, in an attempt to reverse the creeping weight loss, it's agreed that Ben will increase his calorie intake by an extra 200 a day. On this occasion my incessant nagging has obviously worked. Ben reluctantly agrees. I say that if he continues to lose weight then I want to take back control of the eating. Thankfully this is agreed, too.

Every four sessions we all get together for a family session: Ben, Sarah, Linda and me. "I think Ben can continue taking charge of his own eating for another week," Linda pipes up at the next session before I can object. Ben has gained 0.1kg.

The demon spends the rest of the day punishing me for the "massive" weight gain. And, of course, it has no intention of allowing Ben to eat an extra 200 calories a day.

CAMHS SUGGEST IT MIGHT be a good idea to send us on a series of group sessions aimed at helping Ben to manage his anxiety. The venue is the CAMHS in-patient unit.

One hot sunny day in June Ben and I arrive at the unit - a large 18th century former country house surrounded by high fences and locked gates. Either they don't want anyone to get in, or they don't want anyone to get out in a hurry. It is like Fort Knox.

We join the others at a large table in the canteen. Most of the other teens on the course appear to have varying degrees of OCD; Ben is the only one with an eating disorder. My heart sinks as a sandwich lunch is brought over: plate after plate of unappetising NHS sandwiches. Then they place an enormous plate of fried potato chips on the table together with some fruit juice and crisps. While the others tuck in, Ben just sits there looking miserable. He takes a couple of reluctant bites from a sandwich, but apart from that he doesn't eat a thing.

I glance around the room. Apart from us it's empty. Well, almost empty. Over on the left I notice a girl with matted greasy hair wearing a bathrobe over some jeans, sitting in front of some food. Someone is sitting beside her, presumably supervising. The girl is skin and bone. If I think Ben looks bad then she looks a thousand times worse. She just sits there, picking at the food, looking so very ill, her gaunt face completely expressionless as her companion encourages her to eat.

I don't want Ben to end up like this, I scream inside, moving my eyes from the skeletal girl to Ben who, on my right, doesn't want to eat either. But, to be honest, those bland NHS sandwiches look about as appetising as cardboard.

One of the course leaders walks over to the end of the table where we are sitting. She's aware that Ben has anorexia. "I'm sorry," she says, "I should have realised that Ben will require special lunch arrangements. What is your treatment team instructing you to do at the moment?"

"Er, nothing really," I reply. All we seem to be doing is muddling through a Ben-tweaked eating plan that is failing by the day.

We manage three sessions of the anxiety group - and three sandwich lunches which Ben doesn't eat - until both of us decide it's a waste of time. At each session we're split into two groups: parents and teenagers. A young woman with vermillion hair and hippy clothes takes the parents into another room, hands round chewing gum and talks about the ins and outs of anxiety and OCD. Later we join the teenagers down the corridor for an anxiety-busting meditation exercise.

What on earth are we doing here? Ben is wondering the same. The Real Ben, not the demon. We quit after the third session like a couple of conspirators, giggling because the sessions seem so absurd. For a while I feel as if I have the old Ben back - the close team we've always been, fuelled by Ben's ironic philosophical take on life which never fails to make me smile.

17

alice

BEING PART OF THE NORMAL world as it goes on around you is unsettling. Most of the time I feel as if I'm in a bubble looking out - or in a parallel universe. I'm here, but I'm not here. It is quite surreal. And only a few people have any idea what's going on. When I leave the house the neighbours say hello. Kids cycle up and down the road. The lady over the road takes her poodle for a walk. Life goes on as normal. But inside the house it's a very different story.

I've already had a quiet word with the woman next door. "I just thought I'd better explain what's going on if you hear a lot of banging and shouting. Ben isn't well; he has anorexia…" I've no idea how to explain why anorexia can mean banging and shouting, so I just leave it at that. She makes sympathetic noises, nodding her head.

One day our Indian neighbours invite us to their son's 21st birthday party in the local village hall. Predictably Ben starves himself all day "to make room for all the curries swimming in ghee". As expected, the tables are laden with mouth-watering food; the whole focus is on food. "Tuck in!" our genial host exclaims, slapping Ben on the back jovially. "You look as if you could do with a square meal inside you!" followed by "Come on, eat up, there's plenty more where that came from!" as Ben sits in front of his plate, picking at the food miserably.

Around us the party is in full swing. A constant supply of drinks and food… it's foodie heaven. The cooking smells are to die for and the kaleidoscope of tastes is incredible. I want to eat until I can't eat any more.

But I scarcely eat a thing.

I can't eat because of what Ben is going through. As he sits there miserably, turning down offers of drinks and yet more food, Paul and I sit there miserably, too, wanting to go home. In the end we bid an early goodbye to our baffled hosts who continue to party into the night.

Following the birthday party, the demon continues to rage. "Will you promise me something, Ben?" I ask, feeling as if I'm being ground into the earth and stamped on. "When you're a man and you're through this - and you look back and realise how much you hurt me and your dad - will you come back and say sorry?" I can't help myself; the damaging words just spill out.

Ben responds by bashing around the house, yelling and swearing. And, in the meantime, it looks as if he's still losing weight. I feel as if we're on a nightmarish merry-go-round where we keep returning to the same point. I feel as if we're not making any progress at all.

The next day I produce a chicken and avocado sandwich for lunch. Pork meatballs with parmesan cheese are on the evening menu. The demon explodes. Bang, crash, slam! Animal howling, skull bashing. In the end I have to phone Paul to get him to calm Ben down. "I'm taking back full control of your eating!" I threaten, "From tomorrow. No arguments."

"F*ck off!" spits the demon. "I won't f*cking do it. I won't f*cking eat anything. You're f*cking ruining my life! "

AT THIS TIME I'M STILL GOING to church most Sundays with Sue, but I'm feeling more and more disconnected with everyone. I'm finding it hard to engage in small talk - you know, when people smile and ask how you are… "Very well, thank you!" I lie, longing to say: *Well to be truthful, I feel cr*p. In fact I've never felt this cr*p in all my life.* But

I very much doubt if that's the kind of thing they want to hear at their cosy Sunday morning church service.

One Sunday the vicar's talking about the miracle of family life - the importance of having a close and loving environment in which to bring up children. The younger kids are sitting on the floor at the front eagerly waving their hands in the air whenever the vicar asks a question. Behind them, proud parents and grandparents are chuckling at their answers. On this June morning I vividly remember Ben when he was this age, when he'd sit cross-legged at the front of the school Christmas carol service, held in a local church. And the time he played a king in the nativity play and made everyone roar with laughter as he stormed up to the baby Jesus with a face like thunder and hurled his gift at the manger. Meanwhile a little fluffy "sheep" burst into floods of tears and had to be consoled by his mum.

As the service goes on, I notice a couple sitting opposite us. The dad is cradling a new born baby, his face a picture of emotion as he plays with the tiny fingers and toes. What does the future hold for this family, I wonder? Will that little baby grow up big and strong like every parent hopes and prays?

Seeing a new family like this always affects me. Even though it's June, I'm instantly transported back to Christmas again - Christmas Eve 1993. I'm lying in a hospital bed, battered, bruised and sore from giving birth the day before. Beside me, snug in his crib, his eyes trying to focus on me, lies my very own Christmas baby. I gazed in awe and wonder at this tiny being, overwhelmed by the force of maternal emotions that are avalanching down on me…

The sound of the church organ jolts me back to the present. I have no idea which line it is in the final hymn that sets me off, but suddenly I can't stop myself. Right there, in public, in the midst of a congregation I scarcely know, tears are streaming down my face. I am so embarrassed I push past the shocked, staring faces in my pew and flee outside into the fresh air where I continue to sob my eyes out.

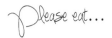

In a flash Sue is there beside me, giving me a hug and calming me down. "I sensed you were finding it difficult," she says. But I want to flee to my car before the congregation leaves the building.

I drive home and face the chaos which the demon has created while I've been out. Paul and I end up having an almighty row. Paul accuses me of being a "control freak" in the way I'm desperately trying to manage Ben's illness. I'm dazed. I almost wonder if he's right and I've completely lost the plot.

Meanwhile Ben is still losing weight. I arrange to see Sarah again in private. I tell her I'm worried and want to take back control of Ben's eating. But Sarah feels that he's doing well and the general trend is positive. She explains that Ben feels in control at what is a very out-of-control time for him. If Ben continues to lose weight then, yes, something may need to be done.

Back home I begin to carefully monitor Ben's intake. Not surprisingly he's been cheating. He hasn't been eating anywhere near the number of calories he's supposed to be consuming. The demon goes crazy when I challenge him about it.

"If you haven't put on weight by September then you won't be going into the sixth form," I threaten, knowing that the Real Ben's ultimate goal is to go to university.

"In that case I won't go back to school ever again," he yells. "I don't need to put on weight. I don't see why I *have* to put on weight, and CAMHS agree with me. It's you that's trying to make me fat. You should listen to them; they're the professionals, not you!" I feel as if I'm responsible for some kind of warped child abuse.

A couple of years later when I'm writing this book Ben tells me that he thought I was trying to make him fat "by mistake", that I simply didn't understand how much food he really needed. "I felt I was fine at the weight I was," he says.

"And every time you lost weight, you felt fine at the new level," I remind him. "And so on... Down and down and down..."

THE HEADMASTER'S PLAN for sitting the rest of the GCSE exams separately works splendidly. And because there's no contact with his peers, Ben's stress levels are reduced. As a result he does really well, surprisingly well when you consider that he's spent the past few months studying at home without any formal tutoring.

We're also making good progress with Alice, the dietician, who we see every three weeks. She's busy working on Ben's fear foods, primarily fats, walking him through the scientific evidence for including fat in a daily diet and gradually introducing one fatty fear food after another. One week it might be chocolate, the next it might be cake.

She calls these "tests" so it doesn't frighten him too much. The latest "test" is the proposal to move from skimmed milk to semi-skimmed. Ideally we want him to go for full-cream milk, but Ben breaks down sobbing at the prospect of semi-skimmed. So, for the time being, we'll have to compromise with orange top: a half-way-house between skimmed and semi-skimmed. Crazy, I know, but this is the kind of minutiae that can send someone with anorexia into a frenzy.

I'm happy to go along with the switch to orange top if I can see progress. The snail-like move from one type of milk to another is, in my eyes, progress, no matter how small. Yet very quickly I'm aware that Ben is consuming less milk than before the switchover. Orange top is proving a step too far and before long we're back to skimmed.

Whenever Ben resists these "tests" set by Alice, I gently remind him of the dietetic evidence. Absurdly I even spend a few days adding up the different fats he's been consuming to prove to him that he's still well within the UK government's safe limits. Boy, it takes a lot of time and energy; but it seems to be working. I've managed to get him to eat chocolate hazelnut spread and flapjacks.

Of course he and I can't count fats and calories forever, it's too artificial. But isn't our whole world artificial these days? In the real world strapping teenage boys eat their parents out of house and home. They wouldn't know - or care - what a calorie or fat unit was if it hit them in the face. Nor would they break down into noisy sobbing at the thought of drinking a milkshake made from semi-skimmed milk.

ONE DAY ALICE SAYS SHE has some bad news. Her funding is being withdrawn. We'll have one final session with her and then that will be that. "And, anyway," she says, "the general feeling is that Ben no longer needs dietetic support".

I'm so shocked I burst into tears. I can't help it. I feel as if everything we've achieved with Alice has been scuppered, as if we're on an elastic lead, plodding slowly towards our destination when - ping! - the elastic pulls us right back to where we were.

Later this turns into anger at The System. "And this on an evening when Ben is refusing to eat his supper, any of it, because the onion I'm using in the pasta sauce is 'swimming in oil'," I wail to Sue over the phone. "And yesterday he cut off all the fat from a slice of bacon, leaving only a tiny bit of meat. This is the boy that our local NHS has decided no longer needs a dietician!"

"Well you know what to do," she says. "Do what I've been doing with breast cancer awareness and write letters to important people - lots of letters to lots of people!"

So I spend the next few days drafting out letters. I complain, I phone official NHS people, I plead with the Commissioners, even the Head of CAMHS with whom I have a long and frustratingly fruitless conversation over the phone - all without any success. There's nothing I can do. We've lost our dietician, just as I feel we're beginning to make progress.

18

the roof

THE DEMON IS RAGING. "I hate myself," it spits at me. "Everyone hates me. I'm so fat and ugly it's disgusting. You're making me fat. CAMHS is making me fat. Everyone is making me fat. You just want to keep on force-feeding me until I explode. You're torturing me! My life is hell - I don't know why the f*ck I'm alive!" He wrenches himself free from the grip I have on his arm and flies up to his room screaming.

A couple of years later, when I'm in the process of writing this book, I challenge him about this. "Tell me more about the rages - for example when you became violent, like if I came into your room following an outburst. Or when you just stood there staring blankly into space."

"I didn't want to talk," Ben says. "I needed time on my own to think. When you saw me looking like a zombie, it was me trying to think, trying to come up with solutions and calm down. It was so hard to calm down with you buzzing around getting distressed. I just wanted to be left on my own. On the other hand, sometimes my thoughts would get really bad - deep bad thoughts - and it probably wasn't such a bad thing you were there."

"Deep bad thoughts?"

"Like the time I nearly climbed onto the roof. Suicidal thoughts."

"Did you ever really plan to kill yourself? Either on purpose or by accident, by doing something dangerous?"

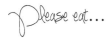

I dread his reply.

"I did think of suicide a lot and, yes, I admit I did want to kill myself. But I'm too frightened of pain, so I doubt if I would have had the courage to do it."

Phew, I relax a bit.

I ask him to tell me more about the roof incident. "If I hadn't rushed up to your room and seen your legs hanging from the skylight and pulled you back in, would you have climbed onto the roof?"

"Probably not. I was too scared of the pain if I fell off; it's a long way to the ground..."

My mind flashes back to that night. By this stage Ben has made suicidal threats on a number of occasions and, by now, I've hidden all the medicines and anything else he might grab in a fit of desperation. But tonight he seems capable of anything. He seems super-human. Unnaturally so. Anything that remains of the Real Ben has completely disappeared. I can tell the demon is hell bent on destruction.

With a mother's instinct I charge up the two flights of stairs and into Ben's attic bedroom. I rush over to where he is climbing out, his torso already on the roof tiles, legs dangling from the skylight into the room as he tries to pull himself onto the roof. I grasp his legs and tug him back into the room until his feet touch the floor. I slam the window closed and place myself like a shield between it and Ben.

I grab him, shaking like a leaf. Suddenly we're hugging each other, the tears streaming down our faces.

"What were you thinking of?" I sob, hugging my beautiful son close. The Real Ben... But - ping! - suddenly he's gone and the zombie is back. His eyes go blank, his face is wiped of its expression and he shrugs his shoulders. "I haven't a clue," he says in a monotone - the voice of the demon.

"I mean, what were you planning to do?"

"Get onto the roof of course," says the slow, low, deep voice that makes my blood freeze.

"Why?"

He shrugs again, looking over my shoulder at nothing in particular. I can't even begin to describe the evening we have after that… I reach my lowest-ever point as a parent. Hell? That would have seemed like a pleasant vacation. "I never want to be that frightened again," I tell Sue.

Later that night I post an SOS on the ATDT forum: "What the heck are parents supposed to do in this situation? Everyone jokes about 'sending for the men in white coats', but in reality what do you do when your child is so distressed they don't care if they kill themselves?"

From Suffolk to the Southern States of America, the mums rally round with support. What's just as distressing is how many of them have been through similar experiences, watching helplessly as their children inflict harm on themselves - or go AWOL for hours on end. One teenager disappeared into the snow in the middle of the night dressed only in her bathrobe and slippers. Another gouged deep cuts across her stomach. I hear of worse accounts, too. By early next morning I have a string of supportive emails from across the globe. I want to physically hug everyone that cares enough about me to get in touch.

At 3am when I can't sleep I begin an urgent email to Sarah which I want her to read before our 11am session. I write that this is a risk we can't ignore. Even if Ben doesn't intend to kill himself, he could easily do so unintentionally. I insist that we resume the weekly sessions instead of the current fortnightly arrangement. I tell her that last night put the fear of God into me. I firmly believe I nearly lost my son.

The next day Ben and I sit in the grim little room with Sarah who, thank goodness, is taking it seriously. But, unless Ben actually harms himself, there's little she can do except thoroughly check with him what his intentions were. Did he plan to kill himself or was it just a cry for help? Might he have similar thoughts in the future? I dread him giving the "wrong" answer.

Another afternoon I get a phone call from the mother of one of Ben's friends. "I hope you don't mind me calling," she says quickly, "But Tom's just had an email from Ben saying, *'Give me one good reason why I should carry on living'*. I felt I should let you know in case… well…" Her words trail off. She doesn't know what to say.

I don't know what to say either. "Ben's been ill. He's not himself. I am so sorry…"

Ben is stony faced when I tell him, not dissimilar to the way he was after the roof incident. Then, without warning, the demon kicks off. Ben goes crazy, bashing around the house like a maniac. He seems to have gone completely insane. I call Sue but get her answering machine. My sister is out, too. So I call CAMHS for help. Sarah is on leave, so I speak to the duty psychiatrist. She says there's nothing CAMHS can do "unless he actually inflicts harm on himself or others". She's very apologetic but her hands are tied.

"Can't I just bring him in so someone can calm him down?" I plead, explaining that I'm in the house alone with him, my husband is working away and I'm terrified. But she abruptly informs me that "CAMHS isn't a 24-hour emergency service".

In desperation I phone Paul, but Ben refuses to talk to him. To make matters worse, Paul starts to blame me. "Everything would be running smoothly if it wasn't for you. You and your cronies on that forum, what do you know? You're only parents. Everything you are doing goes against professional advice! Just let CAMHS get on with it. Look what happens when you try to do it your way!"

"You mean when I try to get him to eat…"

What am I supposed to do? Just sit there and let Ben kill himself by hurling himself off the roof? Let him terrify his friends with suicidal emails? Let the anorexia destroy him without so much as a fight? My gut instinct ever since the day Ben and I struggled through his difficult birth has been to fight. But now I'm seriously beginning to doubt myself. Is it really my fault that the demon erupts as much as it does? If I kept quiet, would it keep quiet too? Am I wrong to question things? Worse, could I actually be driving him to take his own life? All that nagging and buzzing around? All that pleading? All those tears? *How could I live with that?* Yet how could I live with taking a back seat while my son hurtles down the slippery slope to starvation?

My natural instinct is to save his life by whatever means. Yet I have no idea what I should or should not be doing. I take refuge on my favourite foot stool, nice and low down, making it easy to curl myself up into a ball, sobbing into the dwindling supply of tissues.

I arrange an emergency appointment for Ben to see Sarah on her return. He sits there, refusing to speak. He's about to erupt. I can tell. A red flush spreads from his ears across his face. His body tenses. Suddenly he stands up, grabs the coffee table with both hands and hurls it across the room, missing Sarah by inches. Then he storms out.

"Okay…" Sarah says to me, retrieving the box of tissues from the corner of the room and placing the table back in position. "Want to talk about it?"

"This is what his rages are like," I tell her desperately as she pushes the box of tissues towards me. It all spills out. His moods, his threats, his rages, his violence… As Ben disappears to God only knows where on the hospital campus I feel as if *I'm* the patient and Sarah is my therapist. She hands me another tissue as I sit there, head in hands. "Should I go after him?" I ask, feeling helpless.

Sarah says she's sure he'll come back once he's calmed down. "If he's not back in five minutes, I'll send someone out to look for him."

Then she adds sympathetically: "If he's lost weight at our scheduled session tomorrow then we'll return to the eating plan.

Also, if you feel it would help, we'll revert back to weekly sessions - and you can sit in on all of them. How does this sound?"

For the first time I feel as if she's beginning to understand what is driving me: the sheer and utter dread of losing my one and only son to this illness. This, plus the need to be actively involved in his recovery. After all, I'm his parent. I'm with him all week whereas CAMHS only see him for 60 all-too-brief minutes. We need to put every moment of the time I'm with him to positive and practical use.

The door opens and Ben walks back into the room. He sits down. Sarah behaves as if nothing has happened, so I take my cue from her and hide my emotions.

But at least Ben is talking.

THE NEXT DAY WE TURN UP for our usual CAMHS session. Sarah takes Ben to be weighed while I sit in the shabby waiting room. This time I'm hoping that Ben has lost weight so I can be given back control of his eating.

Oh heck, he's put on weight. I can tell by the look of thunder on his face. So, for the next week at least, Ben will remain in charge of his eating, not me. And, as is always the case when he gains weight, the entire valuable 60 minutes are hijacked by the need to pacify Ben and help him come to terms with it. This usually fails and he takes it out on me on the way home.

Sarah reads my mind. "I know you're worried about Ben's recent weight loss and I understand your anxiety, I really do. But to be honest I'm not unduly concerned about the weight loss at this stage and," she says smiling encouragingly at Ben, "he's done so well, he truly has". Ben shoots me one of those *"See, I told you I'm fine!"* looks I'm so familiar with.

Her aim, Sarah says, is to reduce the stress on Ben. She feels things are moving a little too quickly for him what with the recent weight gain and the stress of the eating plan. He's finding it hard to cope and she doesn't want a relapse, especially with our family vacation coming up. "The eating disorder is taking its toll on all of you," she adds. "I think your holiday will be a great opportunity for you to take a break from it, to put the eating disorder on a back burner and have a normal relaxing family vacation."

"And tell her *she* mustn't nag me," hisses the demon in an accusing voice. The demon always refers to me as *she* or *her*.

"I think it will be helpful to all of you if you avoid talking about the eating disorder," Sarah repeats. "Just try to have a nice normal happy family holiday."

"Tell her *she* mustn't mention food or weight." The demon glares at me with its snake-like eyes. "Make *her* agree!"

19

at sea

WE'RE ON OUR WAY TO FRANCE. Right from the start things go wrong.

On the six hour drive to the ferry port we stop off for lunch at a village inn. It takes Ben ages to make his choice: Thai fishcakes with something or other, I can't remember what. All I can remember is that, when the fishcakes arrive, they are very obviously deep-fried. My heart sinks, wondering what's coming next and painfully aware that other people are quietly eating around us. A little girl on the table by the inglenook fireplace tucks into fish fingers and chips enthusiastically, just like Ben used to do.

"Can I swap with you?" Ben asks Paul, pushing the plate of deep-fried fishcakes towards him. Paul says, no, if he'd wanted fishcakes then he'd have chosen fishcakes in the first place. I can see Ben's face beginning to flush.

"Just swap," I say dully to Paul, desperate to keep the demon at bay. He swaps and Ben eats Paul's meal. We finish our lunch in silence.

At Portsmouth we go to the supermarket to pick up some food to eat on the ferry. I've allowed plenty of time because, by now, it can take Ben anything up to an hour to choose what he wants. It's the old familiar picking up and putting down routine. Then Ben strides off to another part of the supermarket before striding back to repeat the exercise. I can sense Paul getting upset. My own mind switches off in the way it's becoming accustomed to because if it didn't, I think I'd die of a broken heart.

Once on the ferry we sit miserably in the first-class cabin I've booked as a special treat and, later, in the bar. For months I've been in two minds as to whether to book this holiday or not. But in the end I went ahead. Then - at the 11th hour - I nearly cancelled. I only wish I had.

By the time we arrive at the villa Ben is in a foul mood. "We've arranged target shooting on the lawn if Ben would like to come along and have a go when you've unpacked," smiles our hospitable ex-military host. "And cold drinks around the pool."

"You'd like that, wouldn't you, Ben?" Paul says a little too enthusiastically.

No, Ben certainly wouldn't like that. Here in the sunny Charente afternoon our anxiety levels have reached boiling point. Before we've even unpacked the three of us are having a screaming match. Ben ends up barricading himself in the bedroom as Paul wrestles to calm him down. I end up in floods of tears and Paul retreats, sobbing, to a garden bench amongst the lavender, threatening to return to England the next day.

Embarrassingly, our host chooses this moment to collect us for the shooting practice. All fake smiles and acting the happy relaxed family, we politely refuse, pleading tiredness after our journey.

You could cut the atmosphere with a knife.

I'd promised CAMHS that I wouldn't "make comments" or "nag" if I noticed Ben cutting back on food. It wrenches my heart to see him instantly going for the diet options in the supermarket after we've worked so hard with Alice to steer him away from these.

Breakfast immediately transforms from a two-course affair into a quick slice of toast with jam, no butter. If I make so much as a whimper about what he's eating the demon shrieks at me.

Nothing we do, apart from going out on our bicycles, appears to raise Ben's spirits. The beach in particular seems to make his mood plummet. The stunning beach where I'd taken photos of Ben the summer before, jumping in the air, his arms spread wide with a sense of freedom that was soon to disappear.

This year he's drawn to the water like a magnet. Here the Atlantic meets the Gironde River, an estuary with strong currents that clash against the crashing waves of the ocean. Swimming needs to be approached with caution. But the lively sea doesn't worry the demon. Up, down, up, down Ben goes doing the crawl like an Olympic swimmer, goggles-covered eyes unaware of - or not caring - where he's heading.

I feel uncomfortable and keep my eyes on him constantly.

ONE DAY I'M WATCHING Ben from the beach. He's getting further and further away from the shore, smaller and smaller, his arms going round and round like a motor as the demon drives him to swim and swim.

Further and further away, occasionally disappearing altogether from view, then bobbing up again on the choppy water. Further and further away…

Suddenly - as he becomes a dot in the distance - I find myself hurtling down the beach, charging into the water and swimming like crazy out to sea towards where Ben is disappearing from view. I swim and swim, really pushing myself. I'm getting closer, but I'm exhausted. Ben seems to have no awareness of what he's doing or where he's heading. He looks as if he's in a trance. I glance behind me and see the shoreline disappearing, the families on the beach looking like matchstick men. No one else is this far out at sea. I curse us for choosing a beach without a lifeguard. I'm tired. So very tired. But I haven't reached Ben yet. What if I can't get back? What if I can't persuade him to come back? What if we get swallowed by one of those waves or dragged below the surface by the strong current?

There is a stark awareness in my mind that we might never make it back. Here - way out at sea - is where it must all end, because if it's going to swallow Ben into its depths then I sure want it to swallow me too.

I'm screaming "Ben!" over and over again. But my voice sounds weak from exhaustion, like Rose after the Titanic's gone down and she's floating on driftwood trying to catch the attention of a lifeboat. *"Ben!!"*

I reach him. He gives me an angry *What the hell are you doing here?* look. *Get off my back will you.*

I try to make light of it. *Oh I was just swimming around and saw you so I thought I'd swim out and say hi...* Mustn't upset the demon, must appear to be normal... *Why don't we go back to the shore, hey? Go and see what dad's up to?* I'm treading water and floundering a bit.

God only knows how deep the sea is here and it's a heck of a long way back to the shore, but gradually the matchstick men become bigger and the water gets shallower as we swim back. Seeing the shore getting closer gives me a second wind and makes it easier. I collapse on my beach towel exhausted. Ben seems to have zero awareness of the danger he's just put us through.

With a face like death, Ben retreats into the beach tent. The demon is in there with him. All around us, life is going on as normal; people laughing and having fun, just like any other beach in summer. Suddenly Ben hurls himself out of the tent, screaming, "I can't go on with this life any longer!" He flees in the opposite direction, up onto the sand dunes and into the deep forest.

I sit on the beach with my head in my hands. What seems like hours later, Paul arrives back from a stroll along the beach and I send him up into the dunes to search for Ben. He doesn't return for ages. My imagination runs riot.

But eventually I see the two of them appearing on the horizon, tiny dots at the top of the high dunes which get bigger as they make their way across the soft sand towards where I'm sitting, my head still in my hands. Ben is distraught, threatening to kill himself. Paul looks like death. Yet all around us the world goes on as normal. Children shriek with laughter, a father and daughter bat a plastic ball to each other and - most noticeable of all - a group of teenagers messes around further down the beach, like teenagers do.

Well, like most teenagers do.

We don't go to the beach again.

I WASN'T KEEN ON THE IDEA of taking the bikes to France for the simple reason that bike rides equal mammoth calorie consumption. But of course the demon thinks it's a splendid idea, especially peddling up steep hills in the blistering heat - hills so steep I have to get off my bike and walk, watching Ben disappear up the incline, the calf muscles he no longer has straining at the gradient.

I have a photograph of Ben as we pause for lunch one day down by the river: his cheeks hollow, his face bony and blank beneath the sunglasses, his knee joints protruding in ways they shouldn't. One day I break down in tears as Ben changes into his cycling shorts in front of me. As he stands there in his underpants, his body looks almost skeletal. "Can't you see what you're doing to yourself?" I sob only to be curtly reminded of my promise not to mention anorexia on this holiday.

Some days we go walking. Ben strides ahead, silent, ignoring Paul and me as if we're not there, his face like death. I have another photo of Ben standing before the elaborate gilded altar of a large church. He looks so thin and lost.

At meal times I have to be characteristically careful about what I cook. Of course Ben doesn't eat between meals or have any ice creams. So I don't either. I can't sit there enjoying an ice cream knowing that the demon isn't permitting him to do likewise.

I guess that being ultra-anxious doesn't make things easy for anyone, least of all Ben. In an ideal world, I'd be calm and supportive, gently encouraging Ben towards recovery, but in practice my nerves are in shreds. I am like an explosive volcano about to erupt. Holiday or no holiday all my instincts scream out that Ben needs to eat more. Yet I'm not permitted to say or do anything. I feel as if I've been gagged. Far from having a "normal family holiday", it's been a nightmare.

On the nine hour ferry journey back to England I follow Ben around the ship, especially when he goes up on deck. While other passengers lean over the white sea-weathered railings to stare at the ocean swishing by, I'm looking at the railings for an altogether different reason.

I am seriously worried that Ben will jump.

A COUPLE OF YEARS LATER I ask Ben about this holiday. He sees it slightly differently from us.

"You and dad kept focusing on the eating disorder when, if you'd looked a little closer, you might have noticed that I was really challenging myself," he says in an attempt to explain the frustration that caused some of the outbursts.

"I felt like shouting: 'Look at what I'm doing! No way would I have done these things even a month ago!' It was unbelievably hard for me. Yet you were focusing on all the negative things. Like the day you burst into tears when I changed into my cycle gear."

"You looked so painfully thin, Ben. I couldn't help it." I remember the cycle gear hanging loosely as if his body was a clothes hanger. Two years before on the Coast2Coast cycle ride it had fitted like a glove, like cycle gear is supposed to do.

"It affected me, too, you know," Ben says with emotion. "I was thinking: 'This is what the anorexia has done to me!' I was furious with the anorexia - mad at the way it'd robbed me of the past year and of my friends. I felt imprisoned by it and wanted to break free. I was crying out for you and dad to say: 'Wow! You're doing really well!' whenever I challenged myself. But you didn't. I needed you and dad to calm down and talk to me, without confrontation."

He explains that seeing us upset didn't help him. "That's the trouble. The anorexia hadn't just screwed up my mind; it had screwed up yours, too - and that made me feel even worse. I'm not saying I'd turned a corner by this stage. Far from it. But I was beginning to want to break free. Oh I knew I couldn't change instantly, the anorexia thinking was far, far too strong. I couldn't just push it out of the way. I felt that the anorexia was 'me', even if it wasn't really. I needed to deal with it. Which is why I spent so much time on my own; I was thinking, trying to deal with things."

I wish I'd known that. I wish I'd had the courage to be calm, supportive and encouraging instead of flying off the handle at the slightest hiccup. I wish I'd had the insight to know that getting emotional about what the anorexia is doing to you, the parent, simply doesn't help. How absurd it seems that, back then, I believed that if I got sufficiently upset Ben would suddenly see sense and snap out of the illness.

But anorexia doesn't work like that.

If only it was that simple.

BACK HOME I'M RELIEVED to find that, despite all that cycling, walking and swimming, Ben has only lost half a kilo. "I told you so," says Ben. Meanwhile he is refusing point blank to speak to me about food at all. "Sarah says you're always going on about food," he snaps.

Ben's moods are getting worse, as are his suicidal thoughts and threats to run away. He says there is "no point" to his life and insists that he "just wants to be left alone to get on with my life, even if that's a sh*t life". He also says he thinks about food all the time at the exclusion of virtually everything else. Before long, Ben is diagnosed with depression. He also continues to lose weight.

I write to CAMHS that: "Ben would prefer it if we made no mention of anorexia, eating plan, weight gain or CAMHS and just left him to get on with it. But this only results in him losing weight. Also, it is impossible *not* to talk about food now and again, yet he sees this as 'going on at' him. We, as his carers, have *no choice* but to mention these things in passing which often results in him flying off the handle at the slightest comment, so we feel as if we are treading on eggshells all the time, terrified he will either kill or harm himself - or leave home. How do we perform our parental role with regards to recovery if he refuses to let us talk about anything to do with the illness and food? If his own eating regime fails to put on weight, what do we do? We can't see him cooperating with any weight gain diet."

I write that "he is not just back-sliding, he's going backwards rapidly" and that "as a weight gain regime this obviously isn't working and it could get serious if left unchecked". I say that "as a parent I am very worried and I need to know what your plans are as regards this consistent weight loss".

"The thing is," Linda says one day, "Ben has to *want* to get better. Until he does there's very little we can do. We can't force him against his will. Doing it this way helps him learn how to make the right choices and see where he's going wrong."

"But what if he never wants to get better?" I retort. "What if he never learns to make the right choices?" *What if he just can't?"*

She doesn't reply.

That evening Paul shouts at me: "You're wasting your time. For God's sake just let him slide downhill. Let him lose so much weight that he ends up on the end of a feeding tube, then perhaps he'll see sense and turn things around." I do wish Paul wouldn't go on like this, as if there's no hope. As if Ben has to reach rock-bottom before things improve. *What happens if he reaches rock-bottom yet still can't stop himself?*

We try slipping the word *in-patient* into conversations. After his experience in the cardio ward Ben is terrified of being admitted to hospital. And, to him, the residential eating disorders unit is no different. The demon fixes its snake-like eyes on me and says slowly and deeply: "I'll never become an in-patient and you know why? Because I'll always be able to control my BMI so it's just above admission level. And that's where I'll stay." The demon laughs in my face, delighted with its clever plan.

That summer, while the world has fun in the sunshine, Paul and I are going through hell. Our anxiety levels are soaring and I've got to the stage where I simply can't cope. I get into the habit of taking refuge in my bed for lengthy periods whenever Paul is at home to take care of Ben. Or I drive into the countryside armed with a box of tissues and some comforting chocolates and howl my eyes out high up on some deserted moor. And still the world continues to enjoy the wonderful summer weather around us.

"Look, if it would help, I'll take Ben down to my parents' house for a long weekend," Paul offers. "Why don't you take a few days off? Go somewhere nice and relax?" Paul is working in Cheltenham. So the plan is that, after CAMHS on Friday, I'll drive down there with Ben, we'll stay overnight and then part company. They'll head off to Kent and I'll head off to a little bolt-hole by the sea.

Despite the CAMHS session going well, my stress levels are soaring and I don't seem to be able to control them. As I drive further down the motorway I notice something strange; my body is beginning to seize up. It's as if every muscle has locked into position. Whenever I try to move my body trembles and shakes in a way that I'm convinced is visible to everyone around me. It's like getting cramp in your foot, but all over your body. If I try to relax my body just pings back into spasms.

Goodness only knows how we get to Cheltenham, but we do, after stopping at every single service station so I can walk around in an attempt to loosen my locked body, hobbling into foyer after foyer like a cripple. I scarcely sleep that night because I can't get my body to behave normally. For the past week or so I've also had a urinary problem which sends me to the bathroom every half hour or so. The GP says it isn't an infection, it's probably stress and prescribes a course of Fluoxetine.

The next day Ben and Paul go off to Kent while I head for the seaside, still frightened at the way my body is behaving. Despite doing everything in my power to relax, even listening to self-hypnosis tapes, my body remains locked. Also the bathroom problem means I daren't go anywhere. Not that I really care. The thing is, you can distance yourself physically from your child's eating disorder, but it's always with you in your mind. In the end I come home a day or two early and drown my sorrows in a bottle of wine.

Paul and Ben haven't had a great time either. The demon's been playing up and making unpleasant scenes. Ben's been swapping meals, refusing food and going AWOL.

Paul arrives home physically and mentally shattered.

20

back at school

IT'S SEPTEMBER AND THE START of the new school year. As I drop Ben off at the bus stop I'm not convinced he's ready to return to school yet. His mood is terrible, his eating has gone haywire and he's avoiding his friends like the plague. School is probably the last place he should be at the moment. But he insists on going. So, with a heavy heart, I drive him to the bus.

Ben is still refusing to let me talk about food or participate with his eating in any way, apart from cooking the evening meal. If I do, he explodes. So it's impossible to ensure he's getting sufficient calories. As a result he's continuing to lose weight. Meanwhile CAMHS still hope that, by managing his own food intake, Ben will gradually learn to "make the right choices". One day he will realise that, yes, he needs to eat more to put on weight and will adjust his intake accordingly. Week after week, scales session after scales session, we'll prove to him that the "wrong choices" add up to weight loss. Just as we've been doing all summer long. But so far he's failed to cotton on.

I wonder how much more weight he will lose before the penny finally drops. *What if it never drops?* Ben is getting more irrational by the day. I can't for the life of me see how the irrational anorexic mind can turn a corner of its own accord. *And what if Ben feels driven to take his own life?* Already he's made several suicide threats.

More than anything I yearn to get Ben back onto a structured eating plan with me at the helm, supported by CAMHS. It's over three months since he ditched *Eating Plan 6* and he's been slowly losing weight ever since. I worry that, by continuing to allow Ben to take control of his eating, we're inadvertently working with the illness. At every CAMHS session he promises to eat more and exercise less. But when push comes to shove he can't do it; he's too scared of getting fat. Result? More weight loss. Meanwhile CAMHS still hope this will prove to him that his "choices aren't always the right ones". One day the penny will drop. Very soon. We hope.

I want to see results. Proper, lasting, genuine, visible results. I just want my son back. I've got to the stage where I'm panicking and terrified of where this is going. And if I hear Paul saying "Sometimes you have to let people reach rock-bottom before they make the decision to change" again, I'll scream!

Ben has lost all his joy and zest for life. I can't remember the last time he smiled or laughed genuinely; he skulks around the house looking as if the world's about to end. He's banned me from preparing any of his meals except the evening main course. He refuses point blank to eat anything else that I prepare. I'm not convinced he's learning anything from this rigid and over-restrictive eating regime of his. Also, he doesn't entirely trust me to "be honest" with what goes into the evening meal. Often I'll find him hovering around me like a mosquito, checking that I'm measuring the ingredients accurately and not adding anything I shouldn't.

I'm still *Big Bad Mum*, the perpetrator of the hated eating plan - the original eating plan that "didn't work". And whenever I voice my concerns, I'm told that "he just needs space". As a result I don't know what my role is. All I am is the person who cooks the evening meal and stands by while he continues to lose weight.

Only a few months ago we had days when we'd see glimpses of the old Ben and we'd be given a break from the eating disorder for a day or two. But now he's on a downer virtually every day - all day.

And it's got nothing to do with me going on at him or not giving him enough space because I've made a point of keeping quiet, rarely mentioning food or weight despite my instincts screaming out for me to take action.

Ben seems to have entered a new, dark and dangerous mood cycle. I'm on a constant knife-edge. Over the past few weeks we've seen some disturbing behaviours. "You're wasting your energy," Paul says. "Let him destroy himself. Let him end up in the unit on the end of a feeding tube." Not if I have anything to do with it, I think. But I feel so helpless I could strangle someone.

I arrange an urgent meeting with Sarah and put together some bulleted notes to send to her in advance.

But today I'm abruptly informed by the CAMHS receptionist that parents are no longer permitted to send emails to clinicians. It's a case of leaving telephone messages and hoping they'll get passed on - or nothing. Sorry, she says, but this is what the management has agreed. *Oh great,* I think to myself, *let's make things even more difficult for parents.*

Meanwhile, the needle continues to get stuck in the groove. "How long do we have to wait before CAMHS insist Ben puts on weight?" I ask Paul over and over again. "And when they do, how on earth do we get Ben to cooperate?" Already Ben is hacked off with treatment. The other week Paul had to virtually carry him to CAMHS. *What if he refuses treatment altogether?* We can't force him to go. So we need to keep him sweet if we want to keep him on our side. I can't help feeling this is playing into the hands of the demon - but, to be honest, I can't see another way.

I'm also worried sick about the compulsive exercising. He's still doing all the usual sit-ups and weights. He insists on going for a gruelling run at least once a week and on doing PE at school. Sometimes the only reason he goes into school is so he doesn't miss PE. How long will he be allowed to exercise? When does it become dangerous? What if he refuses to stop? *What if he just can't stop?*

There's a new problem that's been thrown into the mix: *insomnia.* Sometimes he doesn't sleep at all. His mind whirs round and round all night long, calculating calories and exercises, and working out how he's going to structure them into the following day. These thoughts dominate his thinking.

One way he tries to keep the avalanche of thoughts at bay is to study at an almost manic pace. He hides in the school library whenever he gets a free moment - and he's avoiding contact with his peers. He's actively cutting back on food again and throwing food away. And meanwhile his mood continues to plummet. He seems to have lost the will to recover. Indeed he's in denial about the *need* to recover.

Ben manipulates me with threats of leaving home or killing himself if I so much as hint at a return to the eating plan. Meanwhile he continues with his own version - the plan that's making him lose weight, week after week until, fingers crossed, he turns a corner. But I still can't see any sign of him turning a corner. I'm in a complete state of panic and can't function properly. I'm his parent, yet under my care he risks deteriorating even further as I simply can't get him to co-operate. I feel demoralised, exhausted and very, very frightened.

Day after day I am petrified that I will lose my son to suicide. It's a constant ice cold, heart thudding, leaden weight fear that drives everything I think, do and say. I feel as if I need to keep a constant eye on him in case he does something dangerous, either intentionally or unintentionally. When he goes out running I'm terrified that someone will make fun of him and trigger a suicidal reaction - at least twice some idiot's shouted "Run, fat boy, run!" as Ben's dragged his skeletal frame around the local streets. Of course to Ben their jibes "prove" that he is indeed fat. I could throttle them.

I hoover up anything potentially harmful: knives, scissors and medication. I start to worry about other potentially dangerous items around the home. I've already locked the upstairs windows and hidden the keys. And I'm terrified that if he doesn't take his own life then he'll leave home and disappear into the ether. Or he'll lose his life as a result of starvation or heart failure. Already he's back to the same weight he was in January - the month when his pulse rate plummeted to 29 - and it's now September, eight months on.

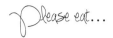

I'm constantly walking on eggshells, trying to avoid setting off the demon. Usually I fail. Like the day Ben discovers he's exceeded his daily calorie intake by 300. It's my fault - I've miscalculated the calories in the evening meal. To cut a long and very traumatic story short, Ben goes ballistic, screaming that he can't live in our house a moment longer and flies upstairs to pack his bags.

"The only reason he didn't leave was because Paul threatened to call the police," I tell Sue the next day. "Ben won't talk to me any longer; he just screams. It's as if he hates me. How am I expected to support him through this illness if he refuses to speak to me?"

But you know what affects me the most about that night? It's while Paul is attempting to console Ben in the living room. I go up to Ben's bedroom where his packed rucksack is propped up on the bed. I sit down beside it, unzip it and look inside.

Neatly folded pyjamas and underpants… his iPod… his wallet… a change of clothes… not much different, really, from the way he'd pack for a family holiday. Then I see the penguin. Ben's battered much-loved penguin. Since my sister produced Fatty the penguin on Ben's first birthday they've been inseparable. Fatty always came on holiday; he was always the last item to be packed into Ben's rucksack, poking out of the top - just like today. We used to joke that Fatty would disappear on exciting adventures while we went out for the day. We'd go to the beach and Fatty would go in search of fish. So - naturally - if Ben was leaving home, then Fatty would go with him.

Fatty…

All of a sudden I have an appalling vision of Ben, Fatty and the neatly packed rucksack huddled under a railway bridge somewhere in our big city - lost and oh so very vulnerable.

Crazily the main thing that sets me off sobbing as if I can't stop is the vision of Ben losing Fatty as someone steals the rucksack or it's left under the bridge to rot while Ben fades away.

A kaleidoscope of horrific images rushes through my mind followed by a grotesque contrast: a content, happy Ben - aged three - sitting up in bed in his cosy Thomas the Tank pyjamas hugging Fatty and beaming with delight as I read him a bedtime story…

I THINK THE HUMAN MIND must do some curious adapting. I'm aware that Ben could take his own life. I'm aware that the illness could kill him in some other way. I find myself moving onto a completely new and frightening emotional plane: a living hell that is impossible to explain unless you've been through it. The prospect of death or the fact that your child may never recover becomes almost "normal". Yet at the same time you are permanently filled with an ice cold, heart thudding fear.

It's vital that I get all of this across to Sarah at our meeting - every single bit, which is why I've put together a carefully thought-out bulleted agenda. "How long do we have?" I ask when I eventually see her. I'm relieved when she says we've got a full hour. I plough through my agenda, item by item, right through to the bitter end.

We discuss intervention plans and safety nets should Ben lose any more weight. We talk about ways to get him to cooperate, especially on school days when he's driven to eat less because he's "sitting around doing nothing". I want to know how long we can let him make his own choices before introducing a strict weight gain regime. I suggest that the time for asking "What does Ben want?" is over. But I can't do this alone. I will need CAMHS' full support.

I explain that I feel powerless. He's unable to keep his promises to eat more and exercise less. All I can do is sit back and watch while he presses the self-destruct button. More than anything else I want to know how she and I can work together to turn things around - especially with Ben refusing to cooperate with me. He's more rigidly trapped in his eating rules, calories and precision-weighing of foods than ever. How can we get him to break free?

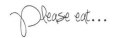

I tell Sarah that Ben can't sleep on school days and is exhausted. Yet he is forcing himself to persevere, working like a Trojan until he's completely worn out. Every morning and every evening is a nightmare. It's simply not sustainable. We can't go on like this.

For the first time I feel as if I'm talking to Sarah from the heart and - thank God - she's listening. As she passes the box of tissues to me, I feel as if it's one human being talking to another human. Not a disinterested professional talking with a neurotic parent. In 60 minutes we cover a heck of a lot of ground.

I genuinely feel we've made progress. I really do. It's Sarah and me against the eating disorder. But how much more weight does Ben have to lose before he gets on our side, too?

21

another phone call

I'M GETTING SERIOUSLY worried about the way Ben's coping - or rather not coping - with school. He's not sleeping and yet he's insisting on going in every day. Night after night he sits miserably at the dinner table, looking exhausted. He's isolating himself, avoiding the common room, has "nothing to say" to his friends and spends all his free periods, breaks and lunchtimes in the library.

He goes into school dinners alone. He's eating next to nothing. Yet he won't take a packed lunch. Sometimes I think the only solution would be to keep him at home. But he insists on going into school, no matter what. It's not healthy, it's not normal and by October it's becoming clear that Ben is burned out.

"I'd lost contact with all my friends," Ben says a couple of years later. "While I'd been away from school for all those months they'd grown into adults, formed new relationships and made new friends. Meanwhile I'd stood still; I felt as if I was *years* behind. It left me pretty isolated which made things very difficult. Also, I think people kept their distance because they were frightened of what I might do or say. Like I might do something weird."

One day he misses the school bus because he's too exhausted to get out of bed. When I drive him to school he makes no move to get out of the car. "Mum, I can't do this any longer," he says almost calmly, looking down at the floor.

Okay, I think to myself, time for Plan B.

"Would it help if I had a word with Mrs E to see if you could come in on a part-time basis? Mornings only, perhaps?" Mrs E is the Head of Sixth Form and, thankfully, she can see me immediately. By the end of our lengthy meeting I think Mrs E knows almost as much about eating disorders as I do. I'm becoming a dab hand at lecturing people these days...

A new routine is agreed. For the time being, Ben will come into school part-time and will be eased in gently until he can face full days. Unfortunately this doesn't cure the insomnia or the social isolation - no-one seems to be able to do that - but it does make Ben happier and more relaxed.

With Ben back under my supervision at lunchtimes, I'm happier and more relaxed, too. And you know what? It's the first time in months that he's actually asked me for help. Calmly asked me for help. It's as if he's finally acknowledging that I am a vital part of the machine that will help him to recover.

Following my meeting with Sarah, the CAMHS sessions have improved too. For the first time we feel like a team: CAMHS and me versus the illness. Sarah is on my side and on Ben's side too: the Real Ben, not the demon that pretends to be Ben. We all remain calm. Forceful and strong, but calm. I discover that keeping calm is the best way to get through to Ben - just like the self-help books always said. And, with Sarah behind me, I find it easier to get the right reaction. Plus, because Ben already trusts Sarah he begins to trust me, too. Yes, he's still gradually losing weight, but for the first time I feel as if we could be moving forward.

Then I get a phone call.

IT'S THE OTHER NURSE FROM the school medical centre. Ben's passed out in the common room and he looks terrible. She's taken his pulse and it's only registering 37.

She wants me to take him to the hospital for another ECG.

Suddenly it's January all over again: me grabbing my keys and rushing into school to pick up a very pale looking Ben from the car park. Ben doesn't want to go to the hospital. Not after last time. Not with the prospect of more blood tests and more needles being stuck into him. I call a taxi to take us to the hospital where we're fast-tracked past the usual Accident and Emergency queue and into a curtained cubicle. And all the time Ben is insisting that the fainting was faked. He did it to "get attention".

"Ben, you can't fake your pulse rate," I say as the nurse hooks him up to the ECG machine and my own heart does a nose dive.

By the time the doctor arrives, Ben's pulse has dropped to 31. The doctor wants to take blood and Ben refuses. "You passed out at school, your pulse rate is abnormally low and we need to find out why," he says, reaching for the needles.

Ben starts to get hysterical. "Isn't anyone listening to me?" he screeches. "The fainting was fake! I did it to make people take notice of me!" The doctor isn't buying it; he insists on doing the bloods, gently explaining to Ben that there's a reason why his pulse is so low. "We need to find out what that reason is."

I can see Ben getting more and more agitated, his features reddening and his eyes darting around like a cornered animal desperately looking for an escape route. "My heart is fine. I feel fine. I feel fantastic. I faked the fainting, don't you see? I FAKED IT!!"

The doctor sits down beside Ben and looks him straight in the eye. "You can't see your heart. You don't know what's going on inside your body. Your pulse rate is showing 31 which is far too low. I need to know why," he repeats.

"I don't know what I'm f*cking doing here, I'm fine!" Suddenly Ben gets to his feet and flees down the corridor towards the main entrance with the doctor hot on his heels. Outside in the open air, the doctor tries to pacify him. "I have to do this," he says firmly. "I can't let you go home, even though you're over 16." He explains that if anything happens to Ben then he could be held responsible.

The commotion alerts the security staff who rush over and insist that Ben cooperates. Ben refuses and begins to walk away. But the security guard is faster. He grabs Ben, turns him around and points him towards the entrance. Ben fights against him, attracting curious looks from the passers-by.

The police are called over. "Look here, sonny. Stop behaving like a six year old, act your age and do what the doctor says." I can't believe that this is Ben, being threatened by the police and getting violent - intelligent, articulate Ben who, before the anorexia, had always behaved impeccably. *This is what the illness has done to my child,* I think to myself, rooted to the spot feebly observing events. I feel as if I'm in the path of a huge avalanche, powerless to do anything except let it run its course. I am the weak mother that can't handle her out-of-control teenager. I can see it in their eyes. There's no sympathy. No empathy. They're just doing their duty because they have to save lives and keep the peace.

"You have a choice," the doctor says to Ben. "You can either come with me voluntarily and have the blood tests done - or I can get these guys to physically bring you in for me to do them. Whichever way I will be doing the blood tests because I consider you to be high risk." He says he can't discharge him until they find out what is wrong.

To my relief Ben finally agrees to go back inside. We wait three long hours before the test results come back. This time it's a junior doctor from the cardio ward who says they want to keep Ben in for observation. Faced with another night in hospital, Ben flips. He begins swearing and kicking things - trolleys, machinery, anything that's close by, before being physically restrained by male nurses. The horrified young doctor rushes off to ask his consultant what to do. Meanwhile I stand there helplessly. The weak mother again...

The nurse takes Ben's pulse. Not surprisingly the uproar has brought it back up to a reasonable level. To Ben's relief he is finally discharged on condition that he undergoes weekly ECG check-ups and blood tests with his GP. *See I told you I was OK,* says the look he throws at me as we leave.

But it doesn't put my mind at rest. I suspect the only reason his pulse has gone back up is because of the commotion. What happens when he calms down? Thank God we're seeing CAMHS tomorrow. Thank God, too, that - as a psychiatrist - Sarah is a trained medical doctor, not just a therapist. She will know what to do.

"THIS IS SERIOUS," SAYS a grim faced Sarah the next day, ignoring Ben's protests that the fainting was faked. "You can't see what's going on inside your body so you can't possibly know. As a doctor I'm well aware of the potential dangers. If I'm in the slightest bit worried about where things are going I won't hesitate to hospitalise you. I won't wait until your BMI drops to the usual admission level." Her words are getting through to Ben - the boy who's always boasted that he'd be able to control his weight "just above" admission level. The word "sectioned" is used. The demon has finally been cornered.

By this stage Ben's weight has dropped to its lowest level, even lower than when I first took him to the GP 12 months ago. "You've got to the stage where your body is literally beginning to 'eat itself'," Sarah says sternly. "I know how much you hate hospitals, but I won't hesitate to admit you if necessary." The effect her words have on Ben is startling.

22

turning point

"WHEN YOU RECOVER," I tell Ben on one of our regular walks, "You will make us prouder than any academic or sporting achievement could ever do. You will have conquered one of the hardest things that any teenager has to conquer. Good God, Ben, we'll be so very, very proud of you." And for the first time in a long while I feel as if my words are going in.

For a whole year I've felt as if I've been banging my head against a brick wall. We'd talk about recovery and Ben would promise to do X, Y or Z, but he'd rarely keep his word. Not because he didn't want to, but because the demon wouldn't let him. As I watched Ben get thinner and thinner, and more entrenched in the anorexia, these talks would break my heart, especially on those days when things seemed completely without hope.

Then - following the latest heart scare - our walks gradually begin to bear fruit. We go over similar ground, but I get the impression that Ben is actually listening. He begins to follow up my suggestions and we start to make progress. Far from banging my head against a brick wall, I feel as if I am finally doing some good.

We continue to walk and talk. We trek for mile after mile along country lanes, through fields of cows and sheep, kicking the autumn leaves through forest glades, negotiating rocky crags and ankle-deep mud. And the more we walk and talk, the more progress we make. No yelling, no arguing, no irrational biting my head off - just calm, positive talking.

Gradually I realise that we're talking less about the illness and more about Ben as a person, about his hopes and dreams for the future. I learn to judge when "enough is enough" on the anorexia front and change the subject to the beautiful sunset or whatever.

One day Ben begins to talk about his illness in the past tense. I'm over the moon. It's not an instant change, but it's a definite shift. It still takes a heck of a lot of work from all of us: Ben, Sarah and me.

Sometimes the demon will fight back and win, like the day Ben goes on a school trip to Manchester for another history conference.

I'm just beginning to enjoy having the day to myself when the phone rings. It's the Deputy Head calling from school. Ben's gone AWOL in Manchester. Staff are tearing their hair out and worried sick. He's been gone for a couple of hours and his mobile phone is switched off. They're wondering whether to alert the police. Meanwhile we're all frantically dialling his number.

After what seems like hours, Ben finally answers my call. He's on his way back to the conference venue. He's "been shopping", bought himself a shirt from NEXT and had a coffee in a student café which was "fantastic". I put the phone down, and then pick it up again as the Deputy Head calls to say Ben's met up with his teachers and everything is okay.

We all breathe a sigh of relief.

Back home, Ben refuses to talk about it. But my theory is that, faced with the prospect of "sitting around all day doing nothing in history lectures", he couldn't handle it. So, when everyone else went to Café Nero to kill time when they got to Manchester early, Ben went AWOL.

But despite incidents like this I do sense a change for the better. A bit like in March or April when you can sense that spring is finally on its way.

GETTING USED TO TRUSTING Ben to be telling the truth about what he's eating isn't easy. After all, I've been taken for a ride by the demon far too many times. I'm trying desperately to believe him, but it doesn't always work.

One evening it comes to a head.

"Do you trust me enough to know that I'm eating what I say I'm eating?" Ben asks me. "That I want to show you that, yes, I can put on weight and recover?"

He can see I'm not convinced and he takes it personally. Then Paul comes back home and the three of us end up having an almighty row: Ben and Paul versus me.

Paul says I need to give Ben a chance to prove that he's on our side now. But I just can't allow myself to relax; I've been hoodwinked too many times. I've seen too many false summits only to be hurled back into the valley to start all over again. I storm off to my bedroom. It's not a good ending to the evening.

"Please let me prove that you can trust me," Ben says to a calmer me the following day, "That we can work on this together rather than fighting each other."

I reluctantly agree to give it a go.

MY BIRTHDAY IN MID-OCTOBER dawns bright, warm and sunny. Ben suggests we get a special lunch from Marks & Spencer and I'm astonished at the speed with which he makes his selection. There's none of the picking stuff up and putting it down. He just chooses something. Then we pay for it, go home and eat.

That afternoon I sit in our sunny conservatory basking in the glow of moving forwards. For the first time in months I feel as if I'm getting my son back.

That evening Ben and I go to Pizza Express. It's the first time we've ventured there since the infamous theatre outing earlier in the year. The grin on my face is 10 miles wide as Ben picks a pizza off the menu without difficulty and a glass of white wine, and proceeds to tuck in. No-one glancing at our little table by the window would ever guess that anything was amiss. And the icing on the cake comes when Ben orders - and eats - a sumptuous desert of frozen yoghurt, fruit and chocolate.

We're relaxed, we're chatting and we're having fun. I'm in seventh heaven. It's the best birthday present I've ever had. I don't walk home, I float on air.

DESPITE TURNING A CORNER attitude-wise, Ben still fails to gain any weight. Although, to all intents and purposes, he's working with us I am under no illusions that it's going to be a quick fix.

Ben is still terrified of getting fat. Just a few extra calories or calories from a fear food like chocolate or pastry could - in his eyes - send him hurtling towards obesity. CAMHS want him to gain around half a kilo a week, in line with the NICE guidelines (National Institute of Clinical Excellence). But his weight just isn't increasing, despite the fact that we now trust Ben to be eating what he claims to be eating. He clearly needs to be eating more, but something inside him is preventing him from doing this.

We still have "off" days when Ben (or, rather, the demon) rebels, but the difference is that, in general, we're working as a team. At last Ben feels he can talk to me about what's going on inside his head rather than bottling it up.

Yes, he still gets depressed. He's still very lonely and dependent on us for his social life which isn't the way it should be when your son is approaching 17. So there's a lot of pressure on my part to keep him occupied and keep his mood up, which is one of the reasons why we go on so many walks.

I'm worried that Ben still isn't socialising - and we discuss it at CAMHS. "Would you like us to go into school, meet with some of your friends and talk about what's been going on?" Sarah and Linda offer in early November. "We'll explain all about eating disorders and talk about why, now you're on the mend, you're keen to get back into the swing of things. But we'd be very discreet and we wouldn't discuss anything you didn't want us to."

So this is what they do and at the next CAMHS session they report back. Ben and I are waiting with bated breath.

"You've a lot of friends that really care about you, Ben," Sarah says. "They don't just like you, they admire you - and they were all keen to know what they could do to help."

"I just want people to stop treating me as if I'm odd," Ben responds. "You know, keeping me at arm's length and acting as if they're feeling sorry for me or sympathetic. I want to be treated like a normal guy."

After the meeting with Sarah and Linda, Ben's friends try hard to woo him back into their social group. But Ben still finds it difficult to integrate claiming that "instead of being treated like a mate I'm just an acquaintance. People are being nice for nice sake. There's nothing wrong with that but it's nice to have real friends, real mates you can get on with".

THE ROAD TO RECOVERY is painfully slow, often coming to a halt for weeks before gently getting back into gear again. But at least Ben doesn't slide backwards. This time it really seems as if he is determined to make a go of it, as if he's found new strength from somewhere. "The anorexia has already stolen a year from my life," he says earnestly on one of our walks, "I'm not letting it steal any more!"

Of course the demon tries its level best to sabotage Ben's slow progress. Take the insomnia, for example, the sleepless nights that no-one seems to be able to fix. And he's still not gaining weight.

Then there's the compulsive exercising. Ben still feels a constant need to purge calories out of his system by running, doing press-ups or whatever. At virtually every CAMHS session Ben agrees to do less exercise and eat more food. But it doesn't happen; if anything he's exercising more than ever. One night I catch him in the kitchen punching the air with his fists. "I just can't help it, mum," he sobs against my shoulder.

Whenever he eats a little more than usual he instantly feels guilty and descends into a deep depressive mood. "I'm finding it so very hard," he says time and time again, and the struggle begins to show in his general frame of mind. Although, over the past weeks, we've seen the Real Ben emerging, and I feel more upbeat than I've done for over a year, I'm acutely aware that the demon is trying to lure him back.

But the good news is that, these days, Ben tells me when he's struggling and asks for help. We're no longer at loggerheads and I genuinely feel as if the walking on eggshells days are finally over.

"The thing about anorexia is that it tries to shout louder than us: the goodies," I say as winter approaches. "So far you've been as strong as an ox and I want you to build on those strengths to kick the anorexia out of your life. I know you're finding it tough. But you're doing a fantastic job. It's not going to happen overnight. Progress will be slow, but it will still be progress."

Slowly but surely things are improving: Ben's state of mind, his eating and the challenges he's setting himself - like eating things he wouldn't have touched with a barge pole just a few months ago such as chocolate, jam and baked goodies containing fats.

For the first time in months he's getting a healthy, balanced diet. His skin tone and colour are improving and he's losing the dark rings around his eyes. Importantly, regular ECG tests are showing a normal pulse rate. The only thing that isn't improving is his weight. And I'm certain that the primary culprit is exercise.

Exercise becomes top of our "to do" list.

23

the contract

BY JANUARY 2011, BEN'S weight is hovering around the same low level. He's not gaining, but neither is he losing which, I tell myself, is Good News after months of steady weight loss.

Okay it's not an ideal situation in that he is still counting calories and finds it virtually impossible to go over his current daily total by more than, say, 20 or 30 calories. But the difference is that he's not resisting. And, unlike a year ago, he isn't cheating, fibbing, cutting down or secretly throwing food away.

But I still can't get my head around why, despite turning a corner on the attitude front, he still can't handle any weight gain. Now and again he gains a little. But then he'll lose it. Over and over again. And each time he gains, the CAMHS session is hi-jacked by the need to pacify Ben and help him come to terms with it. Up and down, up and down by a few points of a kilo goes Ben's weight until, in early February, a further drop brings it to a new all-time low.

Yet, surprisingly, his mood, motivation and behaviour improve. Could it be because, since October, he's been eating a proper, fully balanced diet? For the first time for well over a year his brain has been getting relatively balanced proportions of fats, proteins, carbs, vitamins and minerals.

The only problem is that, although Ben is eating more of the right stuff in the right proportions, he's not eating enough of it. He clearly needs to eat more to put on weight. Yet something inside him is preventing him from doing it.

Ben and I continue to walk and talk most afternoons, and I continue to try to overcome his phobia of weight gain. During those early months of 2011 we trek through yet more forests, boggy meadows and farm-yards. One season gradually changes into another. Yellow and purple crocuses push through the surface and the days get slightly longer. We'll talk about how things are going while I drip-feed the concept that his weight won't hurtle out of control if he consumes a few extra calories or a fear food.

The truth is that, although he genuinely wants to recover, he's finding it punishingly tough. But I have to hand it to him; he's trying darn hard to beat the illness. He's begun to set himself challenges like putting peanut butter on toast, eating small amounts of chocolate and so on - all challenges that would have sent him into a frenzy only a few months before.

"You know that cake I baked yesterday?" he says one day. "I put a whole walnut into it so I'd have a surprise treat when I came to that slice. That would have freaked me out a few months ago; the anorexia wouldn't have let me do it let alone put peanut butter on the slice as well! Oh and it wouldn't have liked the two puddings I had for lunch, either!" Or the two breakfasts you have every day, I add silently with delight.

"Remember how it used to be at meal times?" I say another day. "When you'd go crazy and start banging your head on the wall. What was all that about?"

"It's simple," he responds. "Because I was taking in calories at meal times, those calories had to be absolutely perfect. If they weren't 'perfect', no matter how small the imperfection, the anorexia would make me freak out, hence why I'd go mad at suppertime. The outburst wasn't because the meal was 'imperfect'; it was me being annoyed with myself for being affected by the fact that things weren't 'perfect'. I was angry with the anorexia for doing this to me. That's why I'd 'down tools' so violently, bang and crash around, maybe smash something."

I keep silent, letting him continue.

"Now the anorexic thoughts are quieter I'm much more relaxed about eating and actually enjoy it for the right reasons, more like a normal person. I don't even mind if things aren't 'perfect'. For instance the carrot cake I baked the other day was a bit soggy. A few months ago this would have freaked me out. The anorexia would 'tell me' that I'd taken in 'fatty' food that wasn't absolutely 'perfect'. I couldn't handle it back then. But I can now."

BEN DECIDES TO DO SOME baking. After a while I hear banging and crashing following by loud shriek-like noises... then a repeat... My blood runs ice cold. I recognise those sounds. Something must have gone wrong because he's bashing around, throwing stuff and making "animal noises", just as he used to do...

With a heavy heart I brace myself and pick up some laundry; it's always a good idea to go armed with a "prop" as if I've turned up by chance. I take a deep breath and prepare myself to face whatever is waiting for me on the other side of the kitchen door.

Bash! Crash! Smash! Singing (or, rather, shouting) to loud rock music on the CD player, Ben is hurling bread dough onto the kitchen counter before pummelling it, picking it up and crashing it back down again.

"This bread is going to rise brilliantly, mum!" he laughs, smashing the dough onto the surface again.

Meanwhile I fill the washing machine with the laundry, acting just like any other mum talking to her teenage son. "Do you *have* to have that music so loud?" I ask, faking light-hearted exasperation.

Maybe one day I'll be able to relax without having heart-stopping flashbacks...

THINGS ARE IMPROVING, they really are. It is like a freezing cold, icy, snow-covered wilderness that is thawing out. The warmth has started to return and the flowers are in bloom. A bit like in the *Lion, the Witch and the Wardrobe* when the children defeat the White Witch and the snow melts.

Gradually, as Ben recovers, it's as if new life is being breathed into him and he can laugh again. When I hear him singing at the top of his voice in the shower or in the kitchen I know that all is right with the world. Yes, I am aware that he still has a long way to go and gets down in the dumps every so often, sometimes very much so. But it's not like before when he was totally drained of any joy or fun, like an empty shell.

These days he can go out with his friends without his mind being one hundred per cent on food. He still finds it hard to eat with them, but he manages it. Like last Saturday when he tucked into a huge pizza at E's birthday meal. No more returning home miserably saying: "All I thought about was food…" or feeling guilty because he ate something he "shouldn't".

I remember how I used to say to him: "When you're old and grey and look back on your life, what will be the most valuable memory? The fact that you sacrificed a day's fun to worry about how much exercise you needed to do to work off the pizza you'd just shared - or the fact that you had a great day out with your friends?"

COMPULSIVE EXERCISING IS still top of our "to do" list. I'm well aware that it's bad, but I have no idea how extreme until one CAMHS session with Linda in early spring.

Ever since the October heart scare Ben has been banned from doing PE at school. Unfortunately he's exercising at home to compensate and to ensure he doesn't "put on massive amounts of weight". It's a kind of purge, almost like a sufferer of bulimia might vomit to control their weight.

"Walk me through a typical day's exercising," says Linda as she reaches for a pen and paper.

Just when we think he's listed all the "100 crunches, 100 sit-ups and 100 press-ups" for any one day he interrupts with "I haven't finished yet!" Not once, but several times. School days differ from home days, weekends from week days. Ben is exercising from morning to night.

By the time he catches the school bus in the morning he's already done 100 crunches and sit-ups during the 60 minutes we rush to get up, showered, breakfasted and out of the house. Meanwhile at school he deliberately makes himself late for lessons so he can run from classroom to classroom.

One reason he's still only at school part-time is because he can't handle the thought of "sitting around doing nothing" for the afternoon as well as the morning. When he gets home at lunchtime he pushes himself to do more crunches and repeats these throughout the afternoon - and before and after the evening meal. In addition he's still doing weight sessions most days and going for a couple of runs every week. Meanwhile he can't sleep because his mind is constantly racing as he tries to balance input and output.

The bland CAMHS consulting room feels like a bizarre confessional as Ben confesses his entire exercise regime and Linda's piece of paper becomes several pages. Our very urgent task is to find a way of breaking the cycle. It's a Big Ask. I sigh and look at Linda for an answer.

"What if we draw up some parameters?" she suggests to Ben. "We allow you to do a limited amount of exercise every day and you agree not to exceed this." It seems such a simple solution to a seemingly unsolvable problem.

Between us we devise a structured regime of exercise over and above which Ben isn't permitted to go.

"Then, over the next few weeks, we'll monitor the effect it's having on your weight to prove that less exercise doesn't mean you'll get fat," Linda adds.

Ben agrees to the trial.

The following week Ben and I walk around a local lake. Watching the wildfowl silhouetted against the setting sun, we talk about exercising and how he's making a real effort to cut back. Now he has the structured "exercise plan", as he calls it, he's finding it much easier to manage. Instead of spiralling out of control he now has parameters and - incredibly - from Day One, he sticks to it. And the more he sticks to it, the easier it gets. And the easier it gets, the less exercise he feels compelled to do. I feel like shaking Linda by the hand.

On our walks Ben and I talk about easing him back into school. What are the biggest challenges? How might he overcome these? We talk about socialising and the importance of the friendships he's developing with his most supportive friends. We also talk about eating. What's been difficult? What's been easy? What challenges has he set himself? Have they been successful? We also look at the difference between Ben's eating several months ago and his eating now. And the way his pulse rate is now relatively normal. Most importantly we talk about why a life without anorexia feels so attainable whereas only a few months ago it seemed impossible. Best of all Ben admits that he's finally enjoying our walks for walking's sake; not as a means of burning off calories.

FATTY SAUSAGES AND CHEESY mashed potato: both are things that would have sent Ben into turmoil just a few months before. But one evening in early spring he eats both, without any problem. In fact, for the first time for ages, he actually sees the sausages cooking, surrounded by oozing fat and it doesn't faze him.

In the past I would have attempted to cook "in private", away from Ben's hawk-like eyes, dreading what would happen if he spied just one globule of fat.

"Condensed calories", as he calls them, is another thing we talk about on our walks. Back in the bad old days, at the start of CAMHS treatment, Ben was eating an awful lot of bulk comprising mountains of low calorie, fat-free foods that took ages to eat. 12 months on he's able to include higher calorie foods, including some fats, which makes preparation and eating easier, speedier and much more "normal". Portions are smaller and it also means he's getting a much more balanced diet.

"On Saturday I bought and ate a high calorie sandwich… *and* I ate it in dad's car… *and* I ate it at 2pm… *and* I came home and had a snack in the middle of the afternoon knowing that our evening meal wasn't far off," he says, all smiles. In the old anorexia past, he would have had to eat in a certain place - at a table for example - and at a specific meal time, say, 12.30pm. He'd hate it if there were any interruptions, for instance if anyone came to visit. Every meal had to be "perfect" or else the demon would erupt. And eating out in a pub or restaurant was like playing Russian roulette.

I remember how, not so many months before, we went to a local country pub for an evening meal. Ben ordered a stir fry and when it arrived I could see it glistening with oil. I knew we were in for a rough ride. Sure enough Ben refused to eat a single morsel. Instead he just sat there, sobbing uncontrollably and very publicly, while Paul and I miserably ate our meals, painfully aware that we were attracting a lot of attention.

The worried waitress kept coming over to see what was wrong. Never in a million years would she ever have been able to understand why Ben was in tears, refusing to eat what was, to all intents and purposes, a perfectly delicious meal. After all, don't teenage boys have a reputation for demolishing food as if it's going out of fashion? They certainly don't sit in front of it in floods of noisy, hysterical tears. We made a quick exit. It was one of those occasions when I was convinced the anorexia had completely consumed Ben.

And so it's with some trepidation that we return to the same pub for a meal. This time I'm grinning from ear to ear as Ben consumes a large plate of battered cod, chips and mushy peas without any stress or hesitation. He makes his selection from the menu quickly; there's none of the old chopping and changing his mind before going for the low calorie option and asking for it to be served "without cheese" or whatever. And there's none of the old after-meal blues when the demon would beat him up for being a "greedy pig". By the end of the evening I am walking on air.

But it isn't all good news. Ben's weight is still very low and the demon is constantly lurking, waiting to strike. "I feel as if I'm just living to eat, existing from one meal to the next," Ben wails one night as the demon tries to muscle in. I remind him of all the positive changes and how no-one ever said the road to recovery would be quick. "Things will change, though, I promise."

Keen to conquer the demon, Ben sets himself a whole seven days of challenges which includes more fish and chips, creamy chicken stew with potato dauphinoise, sardine pasta, shepherd's pie and "horribly high in fat" lamb mince, even an extra 100 calories every day in a bid to get the weight moving in the right direction.

"How are you finding the extra calories?" I ask him at the end of the week. "Was it hard?"

"No, because it's not like the days when I'd do anything not to put on weight; now I know I need to and I don't mind. I don't actually like where I am now, physically, and want to put some of the weight back on."

It is music to my ears.

That week, at CAMHS, Ben discovers he's gained weight for the first time in months. Is he relieved as this conversation might suggest? *Is he heck!* He goes into the weighing room in a light-hearted mood and emerges with a face like thunder. He's gained nearly two kilo. Of course Sarah tries to point out over and over again that his weight has been heading south for months.

I can almost hear the demon screeching: *Don't listen to them! All those challenge foods have made you F-A-T and this is the undisputed proof. Look at what the scales are saying... you put on 1.9kg this week, you fat greedy pig! Everyone was W-R-O-N-G. I was right all along!!!*

"Let's not have a knee-jerk reaction, Ben," Sarah responds. "Average it out over the four weeks just gone and you have, in effect, only put on half a kilo a week which is what we recommend."

Then for good measure she adds: "If you were being treated at the in-patient unit you would be fed on a very rigid diet. They would put the food in front of you and expect you to eat it. And if you refused, you'd have to sit there until you'd eaten it. Then, at the end of the week, if you'd put on a similar amount of weight to the two kilo you put on today, they would expect you to continue with the same rigid diet, without any tweaks or changes. So in an ideal world we should be asking the same of you."

But the demon's made Ben deaf. And when we get home, out come the weights for a punishing exercise session, for the second time that day.

So I take a bit of time out, walk down to the bottom of the garden, examine the vegetable patch that's ready for this spring's planting, and eventually head back to the house. Tomorrow will be another day.

On Saturday the demon attempts to surface in the supermarket as Ben attempts to choose some cake. Pick up, put down, change mind, walk away, walk back to the shelf - the old familiar behaviour. "We're not moving on until you've chosen something," I insist calmly. I'm not going to let the demon win and firmly stand my ground, arms folded as if I have all the time in the world. In the end he chooses some cake. I use the drive back home to remind him of what life without anorexia might look like. "You've already experienced it to a certain extent; you've been doing so well since October. It would be a crying shame to let the demon drag you back into the darkness."

I remind him that all the anorexia wants to do is to destroy. "It will lie and fib, convincing you that it's the safe, secure, easy option. But instead it's like a boa constrictor trying to squeeze the life out of you."

But I'm worried that Ben is on a plateau and finding it very hard to move forward. Sarah doesn't seem to have any solutions and neither do I. We've spent the last few CAMHS sessions achieving very little.

At one session Ben becomes extremely upset. He feels disillusioned and frustrated at the sheer snail-like pace of recovery, not just within his body but within his mind too. I'm worried he might be thinking of giving up. What he needs is something to kick-start the recovery, but Ben isn't interested in anything Sarah or I suggest.

Instead I find the answer on the ATDT forum.

THAT WEEKEND, BY COINCIDENCE, a parent has posted a thread entitled Contracting Ideas. This family has been on an intensive family therapy programme at the UCSD's Eating Disorders Center for Treatment and Research. The thing that was proving the most helpful in their daughter's fight to overcome her eating disorder was something called *Behavioural Contracting*.

In its purest form, from what I can gather, Behavioural Contracting is all about encouraging positive behaviours and discouraging negative eating disorder behaviours using a programme of rewards and incentives.

Contracts are a collaborative effort between parent and child. A series of goals is set out covering issues like eating, exercise and weight gain. If the young person achieves a goal, they get a reward, in this family's case gift cards or "coupons" towards sleepovers, visiting friends, babysitting and so on. If the young person fails to achieve a goal, they simply don't earn the reward. So there is no "punishment", just gentle, positive encouragement. Or at least that's what I can see from Googling around to find out more.

I suspect that Contracts wouldn't be effective at every stage of recovery. After all, you wouldn't want to find yourself bargaining or colluding with the eating disorder… But with a young person, like Ben, who has arrived at a stage where he is hell-bent on kicking the eating disorder out of his life, collaborating on something like this might just give him the motivation and kick-start he needs.

Each young person's needs are different. So no two Contracts are alike. Contracts are also very fluid. In other words, they can be tweaked and changed as your child progresses, focusing on overcoming new problem areas or dealing with new challenges. For example on the FEAST website I find a *College Transition Contract* aimed at easing a young person into college or university and a *Relapse Prevention Contract.*

All these Contracts are flexible; the last thing you want when you are trying to free your child from the confines of an eating disorder is to create a straitjacket of rigid rules or routines.

Finally, because everything is written down on paper, a Contract isn't like a verbal agreement that can be quickly forgotten or denied.

It's all a bit like Linda's exercise plan but on steroids. And, like the exercise plan, it could be just what Ben needs to ease him out of the rut.

I decide that we've nothing to lose by giving this concept a go. If it doesn't work, then we'll discard it.

But, in the event, our Contract proves to be one of the most effective things we've done. And it comes at exactly the right moment.

24

points win prizes

AT FIRST I'M WORRIED HE'LL reject the idea. But once Ben realises that the Contract is something we'll be collaborating on, which is specifically aimed at getting him out of Limboland and helping him to move forward, he agrees to give it a try.

He also wants a new Xbox and various other gadgets. So, although I am well aware that money probably isn't the best incentive, the idea of points earning hard cash proves particularly attractive at this stage.

On 20th March 2011 I produce a lined exercise book and type up a draft Contract with a copy for each of us based on the Contract used by the family on the ATDT forum, adapted for our own use.

Everything in our new Contract is designed to provide rewards that encourage progress, overcome challenges and help Ben to set himself ED-busting goals. In other words, we are not rewarding the illness; we are rewarding recovery.

Wholeheartedly.

"Let's do points," I say, getting out the exercise book as we sit down and talk, initially on a daily basis and later every few days or so.

Ben gets points for eating sufficient, with extra points for going over his daily calories. He wins points for weight gain: the more weight he gains, the more points he wins.

There are points for challenges - challenge foods or meals, or socialising, attending school… basically anything that he's finding difficult. We talk about *why* these things are still a challenge and how Ben might overcome them. And we look back on how he overcame earlier challenges to see if he can adopt similar "tools" to deal with current challenges.

Gradually, new challenges become old challenges before phased out altogether as they morph into everyday behaviour. Then more challenges are introduced - things I could never in a million years have dreamed that Ben would eat or do when he was drowning in the anorexia.

Ben decides on his own challenges but I expect at least one proper challenge a day. Some days he doesn't manage this, but - with a bit of discreet encouragement - he'll quickly move on and conquer something else or return to a particular challenge at a later stage.

Ben gets points for keeping within the agreed exercise limits or - preferably - for doing less exercise. He gets points for attending school. The longer he manages to stay in school, the more points he gets: one point for a part morning, two for a full morning and three for a full day.

"Points win prizes!" he smiles whenever I add up the points and reach for my wallet.

One day Ben comes back from school saying they've been studying Contracts in A-level Psychology as a means of aiding recovery from some mental illnesses and addictive behaviours. This immediately moves the Contract from the realm of "one of mum's schemes" into something that's officially endorsed by the mental health world. Brilliant, I think to myself, that psychology lesson couldn't have come at a better time.

Later, in the summer of 2012 as I'm putting this book together, Ben talks to me about the Contract.

"I admit it was a cash incentive at first," he says. "But gradually it became less about money and more about wanting to get better."

He points out that the Contract relies on honesty. "It wouldn't have worked in the Bad Old Days when the ED used to lie and fib," he says. "By this stage I was being completely honest with you about what I was eating and what was going on inside my head. What the Contract did really well was to get me out of the rut I'd got into and help me to move on."

HAVING SOLD THE IDEA of the Contract to Ben, I now have to sell it to Sarah.

At first she's sceptical but intrigued; she hasn't come across anything like this before. But, because we've run out of ideas and because Ben is so keen to try it, she's happy to give it a go. And, from the start, she's right behind me, especially when we begin to see results.

After months of weight loss and stagnation, Ben's weight finally begins to creep up. It's slow - often painfully slow - but at least it's heading in the right direction. One day Sarah suggests we weigh Ben fortnightly rather than weekly in a bid to help him break free from his obsession with numbers. "How do you feel about that, Ben?" she asks. In the past Ben would have found this hard to deal with, but now he seems relatively relaxed.

The Contract also helps Ben to ease himself back into school. Before long he's managing full mornings without bottling out at break time. I am thrilled when he starts to manage full days once a week, on Fridays.

By now Ben's exercise is firmly under control, helped by the limits set by Linda which are now incorporated into the Contract. It's lifted a massive weight from his shoulders. "Now I feel as if I'm controlling the exercise rather than the other way round," he tells me one day.

"What about at school?" I ask, aware that he's been dashing between lessons as a way of cramming more exercise into his day. But apparently he "dealt with that ages ago". I secretly smile.

But the one thing the Contract has failed to fix is the insomnia which is still raging every night. Medication doesn't work. Relaxation exercises don't work. Nothing works. Then, over Easter, we have a mini blip when Ben promptly loses all the weight he's gained over the past month. I insist on a permanent daily calorie increase which is immediately agreed by everyone, Ben included.

It works because Ben regains all the lost weight very quickly. After the initial shock, he gradually comes to terms with it, especially when Sarah and I remind him that we're looking at gradual weight gain over the long term. It also means a hefty reward. "Points really do win prizes!" I laugh as I hand over the cash, recalling the days when gaining weight was a fate worse than death.

But it's not all sweetness and light on the weight gain front.

"Do you feel ready to go back to school full time once the summer exams are over?" I ask him one day in May.

"Not if I find I've put on loads of weight next Friday." Damn. He can cope with one lot of weight gain, but may find it harder to cope with another…

A FEW MONTHS BEFORE it was the table; this time it's the heavy arm chair that Ben picks up and throws across the room at our CAMHS session before punching the wall and walking out.

The trigger? He's been brimming with nervous energy - the kind that can explode at any moment. He desperately wants to be weighed, but the fortnightly scales session isn't until next week and Sarah isn't going to give in.

I sigh as the old familiar behaviour rears its ugly head. Ben is convinced he's put on "loads of weight" and needs to find out. Sarah responds with: "If you came back next week and found you *hadn't* put on 'loads of weight', how would you feel?"

"Happy, relaxed and able to continue with eating extra calories and challenge foods," he replies. She and I have heard this kind of thing umpteen times before; the scales always used to affect Ben's mood for the rest of the day.

Ben is convinced he had a "binge" on Sunday night, caused by what he insists was "greed".

"Walk me through a typical 'binge'," Sarah says calmly. "If I were a fly on the wall what might I see?"

It comprises things like bread and jam, a handful of healthy cereal, a few pieces of dried fruit and nuts and a couple of cookies... Just the odd 100 calories or so...

"So not really what most boys of your age would consider a 'binge' then," she responds giving me a knowing look. Hopefully her words have hit home. Hopefully this is just a temporary blip. And, if not, then it's something we can incorporate into our Contract.

DESPITE THE CONTRACT working well, episodes like this plus the general day-to-day slog of guiding Ben towards recovery is taking its toll on me.

I feel as if I've reached burn-out. This, plus the fact that the anorexia has erased just about everything else from my life: social life, friends, career, having fun and all the usual pleasures that are part of normal life. Also, during the worst months, wherever I went the dark cloud of anorexia and anxiety would come too, whether or not Ben was physically present. And of course, eating disorders are notorious for trying to sneak back in when your defences are down. By this stage my eye is permanently on the ball. I am exhausted.

I also have other pressures.

My 89 year old dad has been seriously ill for months and is in hospital. We don't know if he'll be coming out, and my mum is finding it hard to cope. So I'm trying to split myself between her and Ben.

Paul was made redundant back in the spring, so I had to get my freelancing back into gear. Thankfully he was only out of work for a couple of months. But I'm still juggling work commitments and Ben.

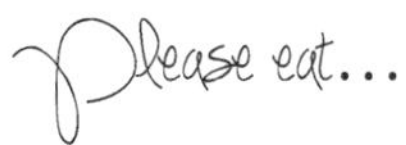

My best friend, Sue, isn't well. One chemo treatment after another hasn't worked. She's lost all her lovely blonde hair and the side-effects of the medication are taking its toll. I feel guilty for neglecting her, and guilty for rambling on about my own problems on the few occasions when we do manage to get together for a coffee.

The good news is that I no longer have to deal with the demon rages at home. I am also feeling far more relaxed around Ben as the eating disorder begins to very slowly subside. But it's still a high maintenance existence: having to plan high calorie meals, counting calories, carefully (and expensively) shopping for food, sorting out school and taking time to do our Contract - and juggling my dad, mum, business and marriage. It is all getting to me.

Everything comes to a head one night when Ben reaches out for help. He's battling with a strong urge to binge. It all ends in an almighty row with Ben kicking furniture and throwing things around before storming off. So much for being the calm, caring and supportive mother…

As always I cry on Sue's shoulder, working my way through the carrot cake muffins and shortbread she produces for me the next morning like an indulgent grandma. I'm cross because she's given me a bottle of wine just for giving her a lift back from her latest chemo session. But I know it will come in handy that evening.

Later, when I've wound down a bit, I have a chat with Ben. I apologise for flying off the handle. "The thing is, the anorexia doesn't just affect you; it affects me too. Usually I'm more than happy to talk through any issues, but recently I've been having my own problems and am finding it hard to cope. I try my best, but sometimes I fail, like the other night. After all, I am only human."

I suggest we spend a bit of time over the weekend going through the Contract and updating it to deal with whatever is bothering Ben at the moment. I hint that maybe this week hasn't been as positive as other weeks and, at this stage of recovery, it's vital to address stumbling blocks to avoid treading water again.

I have a pathological fear of Ben drifting backwards or heading for a full-blown relapse. More than anything, after all this time, I long for Ben to get his life back.

25

rocky road

JUNE 2011 IS WEEK 12 OF the Contract and it still seems to be doing its job. Points are being awarded thick and fast - for challenges, for everything. Some challenges have been completely overcome while new ones have been introduced. One particular challenge at this time is to eat a normal school lunch in the canteen, returning home to eat a large evening meal made from a challenge food, in this case "fatty" lamb mince with onion bhajis and samosas, despite Ben having "sat around doing nothing". This kind of thing is a Super Challenge and one which the Contract certainly helps him to overcome.

Ben still struggles, though. We've agreed that he'll increase calories for a while in a bid to put back some weight he lost as a result of a tummy bug. "Do you feel able to eat extra calories today?" I ask him.

No," he says, which is exactly what he said yesterday and the day before. "There are just too many pressures going on at the moment what with exams and stuff. Every meal this week is a challenge meal."

So I risk resurrecting the demon by saying: "But, you know, you don't just need to gain the 1.5kg you've lost, you also need to get back on target. So, in a way, you need to gain more than 1.5kg over the next fortnight..."

"I only lost the 1.5kg because I was ill; no other reason."

I want to scream at him: *You're bl**dy skinny! You could eat fish and chips five times a day every day for a week and you still wouldn't put on much* *weight, let alone blob out into Billy Bunter! Why can't you blooming well see this?*

But of course I keep silent. Maybe I'm hoping for too much too soon. After all it's only been eight months or so since Ben turned a corner and a few months since we introduced the Contract. Sometimes we find the softly-softly approach is more effective, like Sarah said.

COUNTLESS TIMES I WONDER if the illness will hijack the rest of Ben's school career. It's already stolen the whole of Year 11 from him and he's almost completed the lower sixth form year: Year 12. Only yesterday I drove past the local secondary school and watched a group of sixth form boys, much the same age as Ben, laughing and joking as they walked down the road, each of them looking and behaving like any 17 year old boy. Well, almost any 17 year old boy…

But comparisons like this aren't helpful, in the same way they're not helpful for any parent of a child who is different from its peers through illness or disability.

Meanwhile I'm aware that when Ben is struggling. He's been down in the dumps for a few days and is keeping very quiet. One evening we end up having a fight while I'm preparing the evening meal. He's hovering around watching me cook (echoes of the bad old days), telling me how I should cook the chorizo in the paella ("Cook it first, then remove it from the pan and dab off the fat"). I ignore him except to say: "I will cook as I always cook." But as I walk to the sink, he zooms in with some kitchen paper to mop up the "masses of fat".

When I challenge him, he gives me a lecture on healthy eating, the kind of lecture I became familiar with during the summer of 2009 when the anorexia first began to emerge into the open. I'm still feeling pretty stressed, what with Ben, my dad and so on, and I need to vent my anger on something. I am spoiling for a fight.

Thankfully I manage to contain myself, but I can't help jibing: "I can never get my head around why people with anorexia are so obsessed with 'healthy eating' while on the other hand they are busy damaging their bodies, sometimes quite seriously…"

A red rag to a bull, I know, but I'm only human. And when he says, "You know mum, that kind of comment isn't helpful to me *at all*," I respond with: "Well all of this isn't exactly helpful to *me*, either. I'm a person, too…"

It isn't a bad row. Not really. In the past, it would have spiralled out of control and Ben would probably have walked out of the house or started thumping things. But this time he doesn't do either and I kind of know he won't.

It's why I had the courage to confront him. No more walking on eggshells for me. I smile to myself secretly.

TIME WAS WHEN A VISIT TO the supermarket would take an eternity. It would take Ben ages and ages and ages to choose things, picking stuff up and putting it down, getting it as far as the trolley and even as far as the checkout only to back-track and put stuff back on the shelf and start again. And, of course, the first thing he'd look for would be the dreaded fat content and calories. Today, however, we zoom around the supermarket just like anyone else.

Because it's been so long since we've been to this particular supermarket, the contrast is stark.

This time, there's no chopping and changing, no picking stuff up and putting it down, no checking nutritional content, no opting for "healthy" low calorie produce and no "second thoughts" at the checkout. We just go in, do our shopping, pay for it and go. Job done.

(Ben even complains that the fish and chips ready-meal doesn't have enough chips in it.)

"Take that, anorexia!" I say to myself silently.

IT'S THE SCHOOL SPORTS DAY in early July. Ben's volunteered to help out so I spend the afternoon sitting in the sun on the grassy bank overlooking the playing fields, just as I did two years ago when Ben competed in the 1500 metre race. And, just as I did two years ago, I get talking to Kieran's mum - the boy who Ben beat to the finish line in 2009.

"I haven't seen you around for ages!" she exclaims smiling, reminding me of how she and I used to chat merrily during our sons' rugby matches every Saturday morning. I'm instantly reminded of how we've been living on Planet Zorg for the past 24 months. Or at least that's how it feels. I feel like a stranger returning to an old, familiar place, mixing with old, familiar faces. Some people know a little bit of what we've been through, but others have no idea. Kieran's mum is one of the latter.

Since Ben disappeared off a precipice I've been avoiding the other parents. I simply haven't wanted to talk about our experiences. Not to the "uninitiated" at any rate. Unless you've actually left Planet Earth to live on Zorg you can't possibly know what it's like. Also, there's so much misinformation about anorexia that it's not like talking about high-profile illnesses. Mention that your child has anorexia and it's often met by the kind of reaction that religious cranks get when talking about hell fire and damnation - or some other topic that makes people want to run a mile. Or you get "that look"; the look that wonders what you, as a parent, did to "cause" the eating disorder. I get "that look" quite a lot.

But, thankfully, Kieran's mum seems genuinely interested. "He's still very thin," I point out wistfully as we gaze towards where our sons are talking - her son the picture of health: a tall, strapping, sporty 17 year old while my son is the picture of, well, something rather thinner...

For five long years we've watched our sons play rugby on those playing fields. We've watched them grow from small first formers with high pitched voices to handsome young men. Both our sons excelled at the game. Back in those days, both were *forwards* and both were of a similar height and build. In the classroom our boys were often top of the class; sometimes it was my son and at other times it was hers. Ben used to go round to their house to play and her son would come round to ours. And of course Kieran was always a fixture at Ben's legendary birthday parties.

But all that stopped two summers ago when Ben started to exhibit the first signs of anorexia. And as her son continued a normal school, sports and social life, my son didn't. While her son grew into a big, tall, thick-necked, muscular young man, mine remained in the body of a boyish 15 year old.

And, as we blasted off to Planet Zorg, our regular chats at sports events stopped. Which is why I haven't had any contact with her since then and why it feels kind of odd talking to her again - explaining where Ben and we, as a family, have been for the past two years (i.e. to hell and back) while her family life carried on as normal.

WE HAVEN'T BOOKED a holiday this year. Not after the nightmare in France last summer. But, as July approaches, I feel confident enough to book a couple of last-minute holiday cottages, here in the UK.

It all goes rather well. Ben eats as he should and, on the whole, his moods are okay. We're able to relax as a family for the first time in ages, even though Paul can only be there at weekends because of the pressures of work. In fact it goes so well I decide to take Ben to the seaside for a few days in August.

That goes smoothly, too, apart from an incident in Bath when Ben refuses to eat anything on the lunch menu. My sister has recommended a fabulously atmospheric restaurant for lunch. With its wide sash windows and sage-green panelling it's the kind of interior that Jane Austin wouldn't look out of place in.

"There's nothing on the menu I want," Ben says. Hmn, I think to myself, this sounds familiar. But I'm damned if I'm going to leave the restaurant to find somewhere else to eat. Especially when I can sense the demon raising its ugly head. The waitress comes over to our table. I go ahead and order two meals - one for each of us. Ben sits like a statue, in stony silence, staring out of the window, completely ignoring his meal while I eat mine. Around us the other diners chat above the soft jazz music, just like anyone else doing lunch in Bath. I finish my meal and glance at Ben's untouched plate. In a fit of angry frustration I swap plates and proceed to eat his meal too. Every morsel. No way am I going to leave a perfectly good meal for the waitress to clear up. I'm not going through *all that* again. God only knows what the other diners think. Frankly, I couldn't give a damn.

I pay for our meals and we leave. "Everything okay?" asks the waitress.

"Absolutely fine," I lie. "The meal was lovely."

Outside Ben and I have a massive row. I frog-march him to the railway station, our afternoon tour of the Roman Baths well and truly abandoned. In the crowded station concourse Ben - or, rather, the demon - rants, raves and weeps in full view of everyone. He tries to blame me for why he didn't eat his lunch. "I only went there because *you* wanted to" etc.

"No," I say amongst other things, including why I'm never going to stop fighting until we've finally banished the demon from his life. "It was purely and simply because of the eating disorder. The eating disorder was at the heart of this."

Because Ben needs the calories, I end up buying him a second lunch in a chain store cafe. To my relief, he tucks into a sandwich, a packet of potato crisps and an iced bun as I drown my sorrows in a large cappuccino and a millionaire's shortbread slice, wondering what the heck we're doing in a chain store when we are surrounded by some of Bath's finest eateries, not to mention the fact we've already "had lunch". But at least he's eating - and at least it's "normal" stuff rather than that confounded diet food.

Back at the station, much to my surprise, a quieter, calmer Ben disappears and returns with a Mars Bar which he proceeds to eat. This, and the chain store lunch, is his way of apologising for what happened earlier and of proving that the demon is no longer in control. Rather than skulk off back to our holiday apartment we spend the rest of the day in Bristol sightseeing, sticking a proverbial finger up at the anorexia demon.

That evening I take a photo of a triumphant Ben standing high up on a rock as the sun sets over the sea. The rays have turned the water golden, transforming the derelict 19th century pier into an atmospheric silhouette. It's an image I remember loving as a child when I'd spend the summer in this seaside town with my grandparents. And now here I am with my child - my wonderful boy who's doing his level best to successfully kick the anorexia out of his life. Everything seems normal. Heck, how I revel in the use of the word "normal".

IN AUGUST BEN GETS HIS exam results. They're not brilliant - probably as a result of the insomnia - so we make an appointment with his tutor to talk about re-sits. Although the school is officially closed for the vacation, the building is busy. Every summer the school is taken over by a six-week residential Weight Loss Camp for teenagers. To most people, it's known as the *Fat Camp*.

Our arrival is badly timed.

Just as we enter the building, a huge crowd of obese teenagers pushes past us, squeezed into stretchy sports gear, en route to the playing fields or the gym. Skinny Ben strides straight through the middle of them. It's one of the most bizarre scenes I've seen in a long time.

Up and down the corridor I'm aware of posters pinned to the

walls. I try to ignore them, willing Ben to ignore them too. "Run, don't walk!" they say in big bold type plus other motivational messages about how to make maximum use of every moving moment to burn calories and fat. I'm instantly reminded of earlier in the year when we took Ben to visit his granddad on the eighth floor of the hospital. While we took the lift, Ben took the stairs. Running, not walking. All I can say is thank goodness we weren't in the middle of the *Fat Camp* while Ben was at his most irrational. God only knows what messages he'd have taken away with him.

I squirm. I can't wait to steer Ben off the school premises.

26

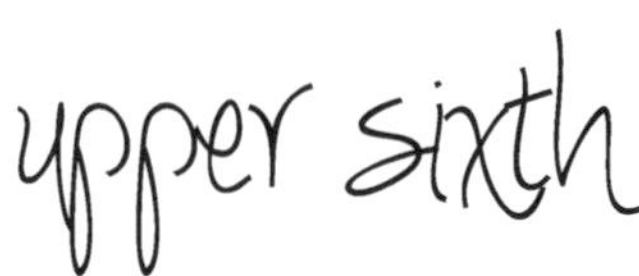

WITH SCHOOL LOOMING and stress levels rising, Ben announces that he wants to cut back on his calorie consumption. Cutting down on calories, he assures me (in a way that makes me writhe with frustration), will help reduce his stress to manageable levels and make it easier for him to sleep.

I insist that any decision will be based on what the scales are telling us at CAMHS. "I can't do anything without Sarah's go-ahead." This becomes a regular chant of mine. These days CAMHS and I are working together pretty well.

Ben says that any weight gain will "destroy him". He says he's "put on tons of weight" recently. I point out that his weight is actually three kilos lower than it was when we began CAMHS treatment 18 months ago. But I'm not in the mood for arguing with the demon, a pointless exercise if ever there was one.

"Anyway I'm off to get myself a pudding because *you* say I must eat," says the demon. Ah, we're back to the old *let's blame mum for force-feeding me* game. Damn the way anxiety and school manage to trigger the demon.

In the event Ben has lost weight. Only a bit, but it just goes to show that he's still unable to judge when everything is okay. So I ask him what he plans to do about it. "I'll increase my calories," he says without prompting.

Brilliant, I think, that was easy.

"But I'll be dropping them back down again when I start school." *Oh cr*p,* I scream inside my head, *why does school always have to stress him out so much, even at this late stage?*

Most important of all, almost a year since he turned a corner to all intents and purposes, why the hell is he still resisting weight gain? He is only one kilo heavier than he was this time last year! One measly kilo. Nothing, really.

Last October, following the second heart scare, I really thought that this was it. That Ben was going to work with us and storm ahead with his weight gain. Okay it might be slow at first, but gradually he'd get up to the 0.5kg weekly weight gain recommended by the NICE guidelines. Yet, despite this and despite the Contract, and despite curbing his exercising, his weight hasn't increased significantly.

He is still terrified of weight gain.

Yes, his mood has improved. Yes, his skin and overall appearance has improved thanks to a balanced diet. Yes, he's been trying so very hard to work towards recovery. And, yes, he's planning to return to school full time. So that's all good news. But, weight wise, he's still much the same as he was a year ago.

So what exactly *is* recovery, I wonder?

If recovery is returning to your pre-anorexia weight, then it's going to take us years! Especially now Ben is insisting on reducing his calories to cope with school.

With a heavy heart I drop Ben off at the bus stop on the first day of term. Ah, another school year, another group of children in their brand new uniforms ready to begin their senior school career. And, in the background, I can see their parents hovering around, trying to keep a discreet distance, just as I did on Ben's very first day. All those hopes and dreams…

In Thomas Hardy's *Jude the Obscure*, Jude dreams of aspiring to the "gleaming spires of Christminster", the university town that he can see in the distance. For several years, when Ben was small, I'd drive home from the advertising agency where I worked as a freelance copywriter, over the high moorland looking towards my own "gleaming spires", as I referred to Ben's secondary school-to-be back then. Just over the summit, nestling in the valley by the river, I could see the school buildings. One day, I promised myself, I would get Ben into that school.

My own experience of state-run secondary school was a nightmare. As a result I'd always vowed that I'd walk on coals to give Ben the best educational experience I could afford. Not specifically in terms of academic achievement - although I was always aware that Ben was bright - but purely and simply for his schooldays to be the "happiest days of his life".

Ben dreamed of getting a place at this school, too. It was my dad's old school; my dad had been a boarder back in the 1930s and was still actively involved with the Old Boys' Association. Or at least he was before he fell sick. Ben talked about "going to granddad's old school". Meanwhile my dad would tell him endless stories about his old school days. Even my dad's illness didn't prevent him from his beloved trips down memory lane. And, from what I could gather, the school still had a great reputation for looking after its students.

So, in the days before the world hurtled into recession, Paul and I saved and saved, assisted by high interest rates and a booming stock market. And, as I glanced over the moorland to those "gleaming spires" in the dark valley, I knew that, before long, we'd have enough money for the fees. So, when Ben won a fee-reducing academic scholarship in 2005, his future was secured.

We were all terribly excited when Ben, aged 11, put on his smart new uniform and set off for his very first day at "granddad's old school".

Over the next four years he thrived. He was usually in the top two or three pupils in his form. He was in the choir, in drama productions and a rising star in the rugby team. He was confident, enthusiastic, popular and extremely happy with glowing school reports from delighted tutors.

Everything we had dreamed about was coming true; the spires weren't just gleaming, they were positively dazzling. Until the eating disorder came along and robbed us all of our dream.

TWELVE MONTHS AGO, in September 2010, I was full of dread and apprehension as Ben attempted to return to school after a nightmarish GCSE year.

So now, in September 2011, I have no idea what to expect.

I honestly don't know how he'll be.

If I'm dreaming of anything, it isn't that Ben will excel academically or on the sports field; it's purely and simply that his final year at school will be okay - and that he'll re-integrate with his friends and become happy and well.

Who gives a damn about qualifications, taking the lead in the school play or wearing a Head Boy's badge? In my mind, by facing his anorexia head on and refusing to give in to it, he has already achieved something far, far superior to anything he could have achieved in the classroom.

Exams can always be re-sat. University can be entered as a mature student - or not at all, if that's his wish. Instead, let's focus on the things that really matter this coming year like full recovery in every area of his life.

I drive back from the school bus stop feeling relatively optimistic. But within days, Ben's anxiety is back and the insomnia kicks in with a vengeance. Also, instead of the old text messages, I'm getting emails from Ben as he sits at a school computer filling in time during free periods, breaks and lunchtimes.

Drat, he's still avoiding his friends...

Don't get me wrong - these emails aren't distressing like the old texts; more a case of "Hi... what are you up to, mum?" But they speak volumes about how lonely he is and how tough he's finding it to integrate with his peers. Sometimes I feel as if I want to shake his friends violently and tell them how much he needs them. Not simply to be there for him and include him, but to talk to him, *really* talk to him, and listen to him - and not to treat him as if he's different, or sick, or someone they feel sorry for because I know Ben hates that.

One day his mood reaches rock-bottom and he won't talk about it. Already he's making excuses to get out of all the activities he's promised to get involved in this term. And he is still isolating himself. When he's in this frame of mind, his eating suffers. It's as if the anorexia instantly recognises the Achilles heel and zooms in to play the toxic friend who pretends to provide a solace.

Ben scarcely saw his friends over the summer because they were "always busy" or "no-one is around". Now, at school, he claims his friends are always "on duty" (as prefects) so there's no-one to go around with. Or "everyone has gone home" or "they're all in lessons". Ben feels he's being ignored and side-lined. Or if people do talk to him, then it's only because they "feel sorry" for him.

When you're on the road to recovery from anorexia, it's so difficult to pick up where you left off before the illness kicked in. What makes it more distressing is that, before the eating disorder took over, Ben was Top Dog in his social group. Now he feels as if, to them, he doesn't even exist. He says he's got quite a few acquaintances but no "real friends" like he used to have before the anorexia and it breaks my heart.

One Monday morning Ben is in a hell of a mood. In fact the only words he says to me as I drive him to the bus are: "Shut up!" Better than "Shut the f*ck up!" from the bad old days, I guess...

As a parent, you never get used to the anorexia treating you like a piece of dirt. Okay this kind of behaviour isn't exclusive to teenagers with anorexia. But when the demon is involved it's a heck of a lot worse because you're painfully aware of just how much time, energy and love you've invested in kicking the illness out of your child's life only to get metaphorically slapped in the face.

And it isn't just that... At times like this all those old worries surface again - my own inner voice telling me that we're by no means out of the woods.

"No way will he go to university next year; he wouldn't last five minutes," it taunts. "Look, he's heading back to Square One." Or: "Why oh why oh why don't you muscle in and *make* him eat more?" And finally: "You've failed. Despite the Contract you're still battling with the eating disorder. Let's face it, you're going to be battling with it 6, 7, 9, 10, 15 years down the line. Ben will *never* leave home, *never* have a family of his own, *never* achieve his potential..." blah blah blah blah...

I try to put the voice to the back of my mind and carry on.

Some days he isn't too bad, but most of the time his mood is pretty low. Day after day after day after day. And, unlike everyone else, he doesn't seem bothered about planning for university or all the studying he needs to do for his exam resits and A-levels. He seems to have no focus. Instead he prefers to write or paint his Warhammer models in solitude. He's even started taking his models to school to give him something to do during free periods.

One day Ben says, "If I'd never known life as a popular social animal I probably wouldn't miss it. But I have and I want to be back there again. Back to where I was before the anorexia hit me in 2009."

I'm alarmed to see that he's begun to blame himself for the eating disorder which robbed him of his friends and happiness. At CAMHS it becomes clear that he's beating himself up about his theory that, if he hadn't cut back on food and increased his exercise, he would never have reached the low body weight and poor nutrition which may have been responsible for the anorexia kicking in.

"There are so many, many reasons why it is not your fault," Sarah says, explaining that the eating disorder would probably have happened no matter what.

At least, as he says, when he goes to university he will be starting a clean sheet. No-one will know about his past and will accept him at face value. Hopefully real life can start again.

Hopefully.

"LOOK AT MY HANDS!" says Ben one morning as we wait for the school bus. "Look how great they look!" He spreads his fingers out to show me. Smooth, healthy, blemish-free hands "except where I nicked myself with my model knife," he adds.

Over the past couple of years, Ben's hands have been in a terrible state. Red raw and bleeding, especially between the fingers and on the knuckles. The skin was always dry and flaky. Even two sets of prescription creams including steroid lotion made no difference. And, of course, you could see the bones and joints clearly under the pale, translucent skin.

Today his hands look perfect (except for the model knife scrape). Not only is he consistently eating just over the required number of calories for an adult man (a slight increase on last week) but those calories comprise the most healthy, nutrient-rich, balanced diet on this planet. And it shows. Not just on his hands but on his face, too.

And, although he should ideally weigh more, it is wonderful to see flesh on his bones. His spine is still visible to a certain extent, but nothing like the gnarled bumpy spine that used to protrude from his back complete with angry red sores caused by too many sit-ups. Those sores are still visible, but only as brown scars which will hopefully fade over time.

Looking at him today was a bit like looking at our cat and knowing you're feeding her the right stuff because her coat is sleek and shiny, and her eyes are bright.

JUST BEFORE CHRISTMAS we head off up to Edinburgh to

celebrate Ben's 18th birthday. I can sense the demon there, in the background. Not a lot, but definitely there. And it gets me thinking that we still have issues that need ironing out before we can truly claim that Ben is "recovered".

Ben's mood is still fairly low and this frustrates me especially as Edinburgh is positively sparkling in the run up to Christmas. But, too often, Ben looks as if he's at a funeral.

The good news is that he manages to eat okay, including a slab of Christmas cake, a large iced bun and a chocolate covered marzipan bar - plus a huge curry and a pizza. But I sigh as he refuses other things, for instance the cooked breakfast on the train, opting for toast and jam instead (no butter). He admits that "not exercising" is proving a tough challenge, overlooking the fact that we're walking for several miles every day, up and down Edinburgh's steep hills. And I notice that he lugs his suitcase up the stairs at the railway station rather than taking the escalator.

Also, he still has this irrational fear that something terrible will happen if he puts on a few extra kilo. In other words, he'll get fat. But what we are still seeing is someone who is most definitely on the skinny side of slim. However Ben doesn't see this… still…

Weight is a sticking point at our CAMHS sessions, too. Ben has been asked to choose a target weight he "feels comfortable with". Some time ago Ben picked a weight out of the ether and he has now reached that weight. This weight is just within the "healthy weight range" on the official charts, but I believe it is far too low for Ben. Thumbing through my notes I notice that this is the same weight he was at the start of CAMHS treatment almost two years ago. Now that, in my opinion, isn't his final target weight; it's his start weight.

Never forget, I remind myself, that it was at this weight that Ben was demonstrating all the signs of full-blown anorexia after having lost a ton of weight over the summer and autumn of 2009. It is the weight at which he was hospitalised with a pulse rate of 29 back in

January 2010. Up and down, up and down, up and down went his weight over the next 23 months with CAMHS to arrive at where it is now - virtually the same as it was on Day One.

This is the boy who used to play Number 3 in the rugby team. The boy who used to charge down the pitch like a steamroller to hurl himself and the rugby ball over the touchline. Even after Ben lost all his primary school puppy fat and developed an athletic physique, he was never skinny. Lean and muscular, yes. But skinny, no. We always used to joke that Ben was "made from concrete". This is why I believe that, to fully recover from the illness, he needs to put much of this weight back on. Also, Ben was 15 when the illness first manifested itself; he is now 18.

The more I read up on things, the more it becomes clear that it's impossible to have a one-size-fits-all approach to target weights and BMIs. Some people - like Ben - have bigger frames. Genetics play a central role, too. Yet, so often to an eating disorder patient, the phrase "you are now within the healthy weight range" means they don't have to increase any further. They have arrived. Period. But, if you look at the charts, the "healthy weight range" is massive.

More than anything I wish that CAMHS would push for a higher weight. I can't do it alone because, as soon as I do, I'm back in my Big Bad Mum hat. Ben trusts Sarah so much that I firmly believe that if she insisted… if she really pushed for extra weight gain… then he would listen.

But he's being given the option of "choosing a weight he feels comfortable with", a weight that avoids additional stress and anxiety. A weight he can live with. And I could scream as I recall the time that someone at CAMHS said that some former anorexia sufferers choose to remain at a lower weight. Forever. As a mother that's pushed for full and complete recovery for her son for so long, my whole being screams out that this can't be right. And, of course, anyone with anorexia absorbs this kind of remark like blotting paper.

So I decide to arrange another private meeting with Sarah.

I show her a photographic montage of what Ben used to look like before the anorexia. I assumed she'd already seen this collection of photographs; I'd emailed it to her via the CAMHS receptionist in the days when we were still permitted to send emails (although we were never permitted to email the clinicians direct). But, it seems, she never received it.

Sarah studies the montage. She admits that, yes, with his bone structure Ben probably does need to carry more flesh. But first he needs to adjust to his present weight, just as in the past he's been given time to adjust to lower weights before moving onwards and upwards. Push for too rapid a weight gain and you risk things going pear-shaped, even encouraging some purging. She's seen this happen quite a lot.

I can see her point.

But I'd rather we didn't talk to Ben about the fact that his weight has slipped into the "normal" range, because - to him - this means he doesn't need to go any further. I believe we still have several more kilos to go and I believe this information will come better from Sarah than from me.

We talk for a whole hour - about weight, about the photo, about the future, about Ben's transition to university and about formulating a relapse prevention plan. But I can't help feeling that it's too little too late. Ben is now 18 and no longer qualifies for CAMHS treatment. Also, Sarah is about to take a sabbatical. Within a blink of an eye, our CAMHS treatment will be over, Ben will be discharged and we'll be left hovering in mid-air. How, I wonder, will I get him from *here* (the same weight he was two years ago) to *there* (the weight he was when he played rugby) without any help or support?

It's such a crying shame that, at this late stage, Ben still fears the sheer havoc that a couple of extra kilos could wreak to his body and soul. He is still petrified of gaining even the slightest bit of weight, despite Sarah emphasising that weight gain will happen because weight maintenance is never going to be an "exact science".

But when we're on our own, without CAMHS, I'm concerned that any slight weight gain will throw Ben into a frenzy of fear and worry. And I'm not sure that I have the expertise to deal with it. Someone once said that these last few kilos are the hardest. Now I know why.

BEN IS STILL TRUDGING TO church and back every Sunday like clockwork. Yet I'm increasingly aware that he's just not connecting with the youth group. He still sits with them in church. But, sometimes, he'll sit with Sue and her husband instead. And he doesn't go to any of the youth group's social activities or meet them outside church. As with school, Ben is still very isolated and it's bugging me.

It's something I talk over with Sue quite a bit. "Why don't you have a chat with the vicar?" she suggests, saying she'll come along with me for "moral support".

One morning, over coffee, Sue and I meet with the vicar in his office. Over the next hour we enthusiastically devise what promises to be the ultimate plan to help Ben integrate into the church and, especially, the youth group. I leave the meeting feeling so optimistic I could dance.

Sue and I wait for the plan to be rolled out.

IN LATE JANUARY SOMETHING hits me like a sledgehammer and I am totally unprepared for it. The sheer force of emotions that hits me as there, in front of me, stands "what might have been" or, rather, "what should have been" if it wasn't for the way the eating disorder had stolen such a massive chunk from Ben's teenage life.

It's the school's bi-centenary year and, as a church school, everything kicks off with a chapel service to celebrate. Paul and I have been invited. All along the route from the car park, snaking through the school grounds, stand pairs of prefects, all smartly dressed in their *colours* blazers, guiding alumni, staff, governors - and us - all the way to the gothic school chapel. Each one of these prefects is a member of Ben's social group - the young people that were his bosom pals throughout the first years of secondary school and who, if it hadn't been for the way anorexia robs its victim of their social life, would still be his bosom pals today.

But this isn't what hits me like a sledgehammer. It's the fact that *all* of them are here. Every single one of them except Ben. And they all look healthy, happy, mature and confident - exactly the way 18 year old students should look.

Their school careers have gone from strength to strength and they ooze confidence. They are the epitome of what Paul and I dreamed for Ben when he won a scholarship to that school seven years ago.

One by one I acknowledge Ben's friends in that long line up to the chapel, my emotions plummeting in a way I hadn't predicted.

Ben should be there with his friends, looking like his friends, behaving like his friends. And I should be making my way to the chapel as proud as punch.

Instead my heart is breaking at the way the eating disorder has stolen a promising school career from my son. The way it's robbed him of his friends and happiness. The way it's stunted his growth and physical development. The way it has completely transformed his life, and ours.

I wish I'd stayed at home.

To add insult to injury, the School Song is playing on a non-stop loop inside my head. They always sing it at this kind of event. That night I go to bed trying to push it out of my mind. It's still there during the five or six times I wake during the night and it's still there the next day.

English public school songs are cheesy at the best of times and this song is no exception. What is so painful about this particular song, however, is its subject matter: *friends*. The friends you make at school and the way this bond remains unbroken throughout your life. *Friends forever...* On and on the song goes, as if the anorexia demon is gleefully thrashing away at the chapel organ, its evil imps chanting the song on loop inside my head.

The next day is the first day of the January school term. I ask Ben if he's planning to spend the whole day in school. "No point," he says. "No point in standing there all alone over lunchtime when I can be at home doing something useful and with people that actually talk to me."

Damn and drat.

It's as if he's completely given up trying to salvage his friendships. Not surprisingly, he hasn't been in contact with any of them over the Christmas break.

"Let's face it, mum," he adds, "I am not going to have any friends until I go away to university". My heart snaps in two for the second time in as many days.

And meanwhile the confounded School Song continues to play relentlessly inside my head: "*Be it to our friends a token of a bond of love unbroken...*" with a chorus that ends with an unpronounceable word in ancient Greek.

I have my own unpronounceable word for this distressing situation, but in ancient British...

Me, being me, I can't just let this lie. I can't sit there and do nothing. Good God, Ben's friends are lovely people. Many parents dread their children getting in with the wrong crowd but Ben couldn't have gotten in with a nicer crowd. What went wrong? Is *he* blanking *them*? Or are *they* blanking *him*? I have no idea.

It did cross my mind on Sunday whether I should have a quiet word with the girl who's shown Ben the most support during his illness. But, as Paul rightly said, that might be putting her under too much pressure. Never forget these kids are studying for the most important exams of their school career; it's not fair to put extra pressure (and possibly a feeling of obligation and - unintentional - guilt) on them.

Bloody eating disorder, I think to myself, trying to get the School Song out of my head.

Meanwhile the mood in the house is subdued. Also, I'm well aware that Paul's finding everything really hard to deal with. The school chapel service affected him, just as it affected me. He had hopes and dreams for Ben, too, and was thrilled at the way Ben appeared to be following in his footsteps on the rugby pitch all those years ago.

But, no matter how much you want your children to take after you, they are individuals in their own right. Ben isn't a carbon-copy of Paul and never will be, just as he isn't a carbon copy of me. Sure, we have some things in common, but Ben is Ben. Ben is himself.

Paul is constantly looking for a reason for Ben's illness - the catalyst that "caused" it, despite the fact that, over and over again, I tell him that it's thought to have genetic roots.

"But there have to be triggers," he adds. "Triggers that set it off. Eating disorders don't 'just happen', surely?"

"I guess so," I respond. With Ben it was the insatiable desire to look the part and stay popular, without having to do as much exercise. After being bullied at primary school, Ben associated loneliness, isolation and vulnerability with "being fat". His new athletic physique, developed as a result of seven-days-a-week rugby and other sporting activities, was what had made him popular at secondary school. (Or at least that's what the anorexia was "telling him" as it lured Ben into its clutches.) And, by the age of 15, Ben was dead set on acquiring a "six pack".

"That damn six pack," Paul says wistfully. "15 year old boys don't get six packs like full-grown men. Ben was fighting a losing battle from the start."

"But," I reply, "His friend had a six pack; he used to show it off to everyone." Or so Ben claimed. But I don't want Paul to blame that friend. Or anyone. Or anything.

So sometimes the two of us feel angry with the illness. At other times we feel resigned. I try to remain optimistic for as long as I'm able, insisting that I will never stop fighting to free Ben from what remains of the anorexia.

But one thing that gets my blood boiling is when Paul points the finger at me. Like the remark he makes early one morning when he says: "That's the trouble with you - you're doing it all wrong."

Of course I couldn't have picked a worse moment to talk about Ben's disastrous social life - five minutes before Paul's about to leave for the office. With exams looming, Ben's struggling with strong "anorexia thoughts". I need to keep a close eye on him because the last thing we want is a relapse. This is what I tell Paul.

So, at 7.15 in the morning, it's like a red rag to a bull when he snaps: "You're doing it all wrong."

Boom!

"*Who,*" I shout back at him, "cared for Ben five or six days a week while you were working away? *Who* had to deal with most of the CAMHS sessions - and take the flack afterwards?"

Over the past two-and-a-half years it's been *me* that's done all the research into eating disorders, read all the books, talked to all the experts, been on the forums and been in the firing line when the anorexia made it impossible for Ben to be in school or sent him crazy, not forgetting the suicidal phase in summer 2010.

It's been *me* that's met with his teachers, *me* that's "walked and talked" with Ben for many an afternoon, trying to make an inroad into his eating disordered mind.

It was *me* that adopted the Recovery Contract, the tool that's proved so very successful, *me* that had to dramatically scale down a promising freelancing career, *me* that's sorted out all the university applications, *me* that has to drive the 20 mile round trip to pick up Ben from school every day because he still can't last until the school bus leaves at 4pm.

Okay, for the past year, Paul has been working locally rather than at the other end of the country as he was during the worst period. However he's been working long hours, often seven days a week late into the evenings. He isn't aware of half the things that have been going on recently, or even less recently, because we simply don't get time to talk.

And when we do, it's the wrong moment. Like five minutes before he leaves for work - or when he's exhausted after another 12 hour day.

Finally I yell: "Well if *you* think I'm doing it all wrong, and *you* can do better, then you're welcome to take over!"

Not the best response, really.

Oh, and apparently I'm "throwing my money away" by sending Ben to university. It's a "complete waste of time" and "he will be home within the year and you'll have thrown £9,000 down the drain. I'm telling you it's a total waste of time".

"Okay, so *you* tell him he's not going to university, then!" I snap, as people do in these pear-shaped moments. "*You* sort out something else for him to do with his life."

It's not a good start to the day. Especially as, later, Ben begins to drag his feet about an 18th birthday party he's been invited to that evening. He's "feeling tired" and asks me if I wouldn't rather he stayed home to save me having to drive out at goodness only knows what hour to pick him up from the centre of town.

No, I tell him, I'm more than happy to pick him up and the socialising will do him good.

This conversation takes place via email - the now familiar emails from the school computer which invariably begin with "How're you doing?" and often end up with Ben asking me to pick him up early.

But today I'm busy, so I can't.

And, anyway, I've agreed with Mrs E that Ben is well enough to tackle full days in school. "Tell him," she said the other day, "that if he misses much more teaching there's a chance he won't get the grades we've predicted".

Home is still Ben's "comfort zone" where he feels he can run and hide. But I strongly believe it's time for him to get out there and be amongst his peers, especially with university looming on the horizon.

DURING THE FEW CAMHS sessions we have left, I'm frantically pushing for extra weight gain. I believe Ben needs a "buffer zone" to cope with any occasion when, for whatever reason, he can't eat - for instance if he was sick, too busy having a fabulous time at university or if his usual daily routine was disrupted. Ideally, I want him to get back to the weight he was before the eating disorder struck. Yet Ben is less than enthusiastic...

"I don't play rugby any more," he says, "So you can't expect me to look the same as I did then".

These last few kilos are never easy and there is the temptation to say "Okay, you've done well so that's good enough". But why settle for "good enough" when you can have "excellent"? Also why settle for anything that could put your child at risk of a relapse, should his or her weight drop significantly?

But getting Ben to buy into the idea of more weight gain is proving very hard. Despite improvements on so many fronts, I feel incredibly frustrated at the bit of the eating disorder that is still very obviously present, making him scared of weighing just a little bit more, making him feel "fine" as he is and kidding him that he is bigger than he actually is.

"If you think I'm thin, mum..." he said the other day, referring to a comedian on the telly who was slim, but not as slim as he is.

But Ben couldn't see that.

Every time we go to CAMHS we decide what Ben will do next, calories-wise, depending on what the scales say. I want to push for an increase in calories even if his weight remains static or decreases by just a small amount. But I'm not being very successful.

Sure, I could sneak extra calories into meals like I used to do. But that would result in him cutting back when he finds his weight has increased, so it's counterproductive.

Today at CAMHS Ben's mood is rock-bottom. I can tell he's extremely anxious. He admits to being tempted to give in to the anorexia thoughts.

"My mum told me that when I was recovered I'd feel better emotionally, but I don't, I feel cr*p," he says throwing me an accusing look, going on to imply that - because he "feels cr*p" - he might as well give in to the eating disorder. After all, he always felt "safe" there.

They say you hurt the ones you love most, and Ben certainly succeeds in hurting me. The session is full of accusations along the lines of "My mum insists that xxxx is right" and "I don't know who's right: the NHS that's telling me it's okay to stick with 'good enough' and stay as I am - or the rest of the world that's telling me I must be properly 'weight restored' in order to recover".

"Well I'm more than happy to settle for 'good enough'," Sarah responds to my alarm. "In an ideal world we'd love you to return to the weight and physique you were before the anorexia. But in many people this just isn't possible. They simply can't handle it. So we need to come to some sort of compromise and I'm happy for you to stay where you are. Yes, if you got sick or something else resulted in weight loss you would be underweight because you don't have any 'buffer zone'. But I'm happy to settle for 'good enough' if you are."

I get a daggers look from Ben. Big Bad Mum who, I suspect in his eyes, is trying to make him fat. "My mum says if I lose weight I'll end up in hospital and die," he says accusingly.

"No, I did not," I snap. "I said that you don't have any buffer zone. If you lost weight you could risk heading back into the 'danger zone'."

I tell him that he and I have fought tooth and nail to get him to the stage he's at now. I tell him that I refuse to let him relapse. I refuse to let him go through all this again.

But Ben feels "uncomfortable" now he's "put on all this weight". He feels like he "did before the anorexia" when he "was fat". He feels hot. His clothes feel too tight. Anyone would think he'd put on several hundredweight rather than just a couple of kilos. I can almost hear the anorexia Sirens singing as they attempt to lure Ben back onto the rocks.

He continues to point the finger at me. "*She* told me blah…", "*She* always says blah…" and - to Sarah - "*She*'s only saying that because *you're* here," etc. Boy, that demon sure knows how to hurt a mother. But, then, that's the demon's job just as it's my job to sit there and take it. After all this time I'm well used to being treated as a punch bag.

A week later we return to CAMHS for Sarah to check Ben's weight. It remains unchanged. So why does this make the demon see red? Not because Ben wanted his weight to drop, surely? Not at this stage in the recovery process.

I decide it's because, over the past two weeks, he's been guessing his calorie intake in a bid to ditch the counting calories millstone once and for all. He's convinced that - ouch! - he's been over-estimating and therefore should have *lost* weight, especially as he's been "doing all that exercise".

Oh drat, says the anti-demon voice inside my head, especially as Ben's mood continues to head south during the remainder of the session: hating himself, feeling worthless, feeling isolated and very, very lonely.

Mind you, this is typical of the demon. Just when you think you're getting somewhere, it sticks its oar in and messes things up for a while.

But hopefully only a short while…

27

losses

IN FEBRUARY THE TEMPERATURE plummets to minus seven. Then, in the wee small hours of the coldest night of all, the phone rings. It's the hospital where my dad is being treated for pneumonia. The nurse tells me he passed away shortly after midnight. Paul and I hurriedly get dressed and head for the hospital through the silent, frozen landscape. Later, as the watery sun begins to rise, I let myself into my parents' house to break the news to my sleeping mother.

The next few days and weeks are a frantic blur as we struggle with our grief alongside a myriad of official tasks. My sister and I spend most of our time with mum, helping her to sort out paperwork and funeral arrangements. Ben rallies round by taking charge of all the family meals which he does admirably. Not a "slimmed down" meal in sight. The demon is absent, too. For the first time in a long time I really feel as if I've got my son back.

Sue is characteristically supportive, helping me to get through this difficult time and constantly reminding me of how far Ben has come over the last couple of years. Imagine if my dad had died when Ben was going through his worst phase? It doesn't bear thinking about.

Meanwhile we have our final session with CAMHS. We both hug Sarah goodbye and give her a big bunch of flowers. Ben writes her a personal card, thanking her for her support. We may have had our differences over the past two years, but we are both genuinely sorry to see her go.

Afterwards, I can't help feeling a bit like a ship that's been cut adrift in the ocean. Both my dad and CAMHS are gone. And, although I didn't always see eye to eye with either of them, I miss them like hell now they're not here.

As my friend C on the ATDT forum would say: "It's time to put on your Big Girl's Pants." In other words, it's time to knuckle down, act grown up and get on with things.

And at least I've still got Sue who is proving to be a tower of strength. Dear, sweet Sue who struggles so much with her own battle for survival, yet who spends most of her time thinking of others.

ONE DAY TOWARDS THE END of March, Ben announces that he no longer believes in God. He removes the cross that's been permanently hanging around his neck. He discards the Bible he used to carry in his bag to read on the school bus. And he starts to eat chocolate again (given up for Lent).

He also stops going to church after religiously trotting to and from that building virtually every Sunday for the past 18 months.

Two months on from the meeting Sue and I had with the vicar, nothing has changed. No-one's come forward from the church to befriend Ben (apart from Sue who, bless her, does her level best to make up for it). And I'm not aware of any progress on the youth group front.

Nothing has happened. Nothing at all.

What we're left with is a boy who is hurting, who feels let down by the very people he was certain would offer him support and friendship. A boy who believes that any spiritual experiences he had were fake, probably induced by the eating disordered mind or what he terms as "the earth's magnetic forces affecting the front lobes of the brain" (or something like that).

I'm aware that his faith is one of the things that's been keeping Ben going over the last 18 months. But now the light has gone out in his eyes and it's as if he's spiritually dead. It's almost like a young child discovering that Father Christmas was his daddy all along.

IN APRIL, BEN AND I get invited to appear on the *Loraine Kelly* show on the TV, talking about the rise of anorexia in teenage boys.

In front of the bright lights and cameras, I explain how things started to deteriorate during the summer of 2009; how Ben began to exercise more, de-calorise meals, cut himself off from his friends and lose weight. I tell her how I had no idea what was happening; after all, as far as I knew, eating disorders happened to teenage girls not boys. I talk about our battle to get Ben referred for treatment followed by the long wait for an assessment - and how, meanwhile, I watched helplessly as he disappeared in front of my eyes.

I talk about how anorexia isn't just about losing weight; it's about a host of other things like depression, distressing behaviour and social isolation. How, over a matter of months, a boy who had been bright, popular and sporty transformed into someone we didn't recognise...

But, all too soon, the brief interview is over.

I never get to explain about the cardio emergency that resulted in Ben being fast-tracked into CAMHS at the end of January 2010.

I never get to talk about the road to recovery - or the wonderful, amazing, awesome people that helped us along the way such as the ATDT forum which was, and still is, a true lifeline.

I never get to talk about how, as a parent of a child that's developing an eating disorder, you need to know exactly what to do, and then you have to do it. Quickly. You have no choice. And whenever you feel you can't go on any longer, you somehow have to find a second wind - and a third, and a fourth. You are in this for the long haul whether you like it or not, because the alternative could be to lose your precious child.

I never get to talk about my blog or why I write it. I never get to say that we want our children to survive this illness and develop into happy, healthy, normal adults. Anorexia has already stolen years from our children's lives; we, as parents, refuse to let it steal any more.

And, if Lorraine had asked what I'd say to people who might accuse me of being a "control freak" or being "overprotective", I'd have said this: "What would they do if they discovered their child was suffering from a life-threatening illness? I'd hazard a guess they'd fight tooth and nail and basically do whatever it takes, even walk on coals, to save their child's life as quickly as is humanly possible. That's not 'control' or 'overprotection', that's love."

But I never get to say any of this.

However, at least Ben and I have been able to help raise awareness of the growing problem of anorexia in teenage boys. And Ben was truly awesome on that TV sofa.

ONE THING THAT'S BEEN put on a back-burner during Ben's illness is housework. Now, I've never been what you might call "house proud". But, as months of anorexia stretch into years, my house begins to disappear in a mountain of dust and clutter. One day, in a fit of frustration, I decide to do a much needed clear-out of the back bedroom which doubles as my office.

First on the list are the contents of my granddad's old brown leather suitcase, crammed with things I've collected over the years: Ben's primary school reports, certificates and other odds and ends, and a mountain of stuff I'd been collecting to form a lasting memory of Ben's years at secondary school.

Pulling all this stuff out of the suitcase and onto the dusty blue carpet, I'm painfully aware that Ben's memories of school aren't going to be good memories. Even though the first four years were really great, looking back at these is a painful reminder of what "could have been"... what "*would* have been" if the anorexia had never hijacked his life.

"It makes it trebly hard," he says, "knowing that everything used to be so good. I used to be popular, I used to be the top dog in our group, but now I'm on my own". It breaks my heart.

I grasp a pile of school calendars, concert programmes and tickets, timetables, letters and leaflets and push them through the shredder. Goodness only knows why I've kept all this stuff.

But I decide to keep the school reports, photographs, certificates, prospectuses, the letter offering Ben a scholarship and other items which he may want to look back on in the future when, hopefully, the painful memories have receded.

As I arrange these neatly inside the suitcase, I mourn the seven years that could so easily have been the Best Days of His Life if it wasn't for the way the anorexia blitzed it to smithereens and left an ugly red scar which may take some time to fade.

ONE MORNING BEN SAYS: "I feel awful because I've just binged on top of my usual breakfast."

So I respond with: "Let's concentrate on what's important in your new life without anorexia, not on what isn't. When you're old, grey and on your deathbed and you're looking back on your life, you will remember all the fantastic things you did - university, friends, marriage, kids, career and so on - and not that on this particular day in history you had a 'binge'."

To which Ben replies: "Not if I'm on my deathbed because I'm obese." To which I reply, in a manner that implies the conversation is over: "Ben, there's as much chance of you getting obese as there is of me becoming Pope."

Oh, and as we discussed at CAMHS the other month, a "binge" isn't what you or I might call a binge. To Ben it's simply eating a little more than he would normally eat. And you can bet your back teeth he'd include it in his daily calorie total, anyway.

So I'm still watching closely.

I'M WORRIED ABOUT SUE. The chemotherapy is taking its toll. Already stick-thin, she's finding it increasingly difficult to eat. She's had a persistent cough for some time, is finding it hard to breathe and she's oh so very tired all the time.

On top of this the oncologist has recently changed her chemotherapy.

Again.

She was warned that this one wouldn't be a bed of roses, but we didn't realise it would make her this sick. "Maybe you need to switch to another type?" I suggest. The alarm bells start to ring as she says there aren't any more treatments available; she's tried them all.

"I must be allergic to this one!" she jokes, "Oh and by the way, did I show you my latest picture?" Sue's taken up art and creates the most incredible pastels: thoughts, emotions and pictures that come into her head. The latest is of a distant horizon with the sun setting, its reddish golden rays shimmering across a sparkling sea.

Like all her artwork, it's quite dream-like, almost other-worldly, and so very peaceful. "It's awfully good," I say truthfully from halfway up the stairs where it's hanging on the wall. Sue apologises for not coming up the stairs with me. "I find climbing the stairs too exhausting these days," she says, coughing again.

Every time I see Sue she looks thinner. I don't like thin. I hate thin. Ever the expert at cooking mega high calorie food, I bake a tray of calorie-laden flapjacks and sticky Chelsea buns in an attempt to put some flesh onto that tiny bony frame. No holds barred - I go for the most calorific ingredients I can find: butter, nuts, golden syrup and sugar - the works. "Eat these," I command, already planning the next high calorie bake.

One day, I'm supposed to be going to her house for a coffee. I've baked some more Chelsea buns - bigger, better, stickier and more calorific than the last batch and I can't wait to give them to her. She sends me an email: "Can we leave it until I feel a bit better?" So I put them in the freezer. They can wait.

I decide I want to give Sue a proper gift - to thank her for being such a fabulous friend. Sue loves scarves. So I buy a beautiful hand-made scarf and drop it off at her house with a card one evening.

"I don't want to bother her if she's not feeling well," I say, handing the gift to her husband before dashing off.

Sue never gets to wear that scarf.

A day or so later I get an email from her husband. Sue passed away in her sleep just before lunchtime. One minute she was there and the next... Only the other week I was sitting with her drinking coffee. She'd given me a bottle of expensive body lotion to thank me for the first batch of baked goodies.

"You're naughty," I told her. "You shouldn't buy me things. You don't have to. You've done more for me than you could ever imagine, and for Ben too. I won't bake you any more goodies if you continue to buy me gifts in return."

I stare at the latest batch of Chelsea buns in the freezer, waiting for Sue who will never get to enjoy them.

"Damn you!" I scream, tears streaming down my face as I sink to the floor. "Why the hell did you have to go and die?"

Did she ever *really* know how much she meant to me? Did she ever *really* know how awesomely supportive she'd been over the past two-and-a-bit years? How I couldn't have got through half of this without her? How, no matter what, she'd always be there armed with a mug of coffee, a plate of cookies, a box of tissues and a sympathetic ear? Did she ever read that last note I sent to her? At the last minute I'd popped it in with the scarf and card. Something prompted me to write the note, to tell her how much she'd meant to me as a friend and what a wonderful person she was.

It was a difficult note to write. Somehow I had a hunch that the prognosis wasn't going to be good. But I didn't want to imply it in the note. I didn't want an "It's been nice knowing you" kind of note.

So I talked about the cakes that were waiting for her in our freezer, and how I was really looking forward to our next coffee, so she'd better hurry up and get better. Oh, and in the meantime I just thought I'd tell her how much she has meant to us over the past couple of years, what a fantastic friend she's been, that kind of thing…

Standing beside Sue's coffin at her funeral a week later I address the crowded church. It's the first time I've spoken about Ben's illness in public - well it's the first time I've spoken about anything in public because I'm pretty useless when it comes to public speaking. But somehow I manage to walk up the aisle and stand beside Sue, take a deep breath, put on my glasses, check my carefully constructed notes and begin…

I first met Sue two-and-a-half years ago. As a family we'd been going through a tough time. Ben, my son, had anorexia. Things weren't going well and I was desperate for support. The church - this church - seemed a good place to start.

My first memory of Sue is of a tiny woman striding towards me, across the aisle, to where I was sitting - or rather hiding - at the back.

She had a huge smile on her face and immediately took me under her wing - and over the next couple of years an amazing friendship developed.

We'd meet regularly, usually at her house - or we'd talk over the phone. As Ben's illness got worse and I got more desperate she'd just sit there listening. Whatever I wanted to say, I knew could say it in front of Sue. And, most importantly, she took the time to really understand what we were going through.

This little woman with the big smile and a huge heart was the most genuine, caring, loving and selfless person I have ever known.

BUT… Sue could be really infuriating. By this I mean that whenever I tried to turn the conversation round to her and her issues - and I mean she had BIG issues to deal with - she had an infuriating knack of turning the focus back to me. But that's the kind of person Sue was. Selfless.

For two-and-a-half years she was an absolute rock and the best and most caring friend you could ever have. I want to share with you something she wrote to me when we were going through a particularly bad patch:

"Please be assured of my thoughts and prayers and, if there is anything at all I can do - or if you just need someone to talk to, at any time - please do not hesitate to phone me. I really want to support you as you walk this difficult journey. Please never think that your stress is any less than mine; it is different…"

Sue always said: "Never forget, if you ever need me, you know where I am."

That May afternoon, the hot sun is high in a deep blue cloudless sky. "Come on, Ben, let's go for a walk," I say when we get back from the funeral. "Sue wouldn't want us to sit around the house moping."

It's a walk I'll never forget. Sunken country lanes, gurgling streams, fields of meadow flowers, creamy hawthorn blossom on the hedgerows… the whole countryside is coming to life.

We remember Sue as we climb across stiles, open creaking farmyard gates and watch the new born lambs dancing around as we take a break under the welcome shade of a gnarled oak tree.

"You know what she did a few weeks ago?" I say, wistfully. "She was bored with her blonde wigs. So she said 'I've decided to go red. Want to see? Promise you won't laugh!' I promised. 'Ta dah!' she said, walking into the room in a vibrant red wig. I mean *really* vibrant.

She always wanted to have crazy hair, but she'd never had the guts to do it. 'It's part of my rebellious streak,' she used to say. 'Do you think I dare wear it to church?' she said looking in the mirror doubtfully."

I sigh at the memory.

"You're going to miss her," Ben says.

"Yes I certainly am," I reply.

28

brilliant & amazing things

ONE THING I STILL CAN'T get my head around after all this time is Ben's fear of "spiralling out of control" and getting fat. There is still something inside him which warns him that, if he relaxed too much, he'd eat and eat and eat until he could eat no more. There is no middle ground. In his mind, it's either slim or obese, with nothing in between. I believe it's this fear that is slowing Ben's progress down to a snail's pace.

I worry what will happen when Ben eventually "arrives" at his set weight. Whatever that set weight is - because there is still a marked difference between what Ben believes is his natural set weight and what I believe it should be.

But, when he arrives there, will he instantly insist on cutting back?

I remember both Sarah and Linda saying that Ben needn't worry because they'd never let his weight "spiral out of control". And, once discharged from their care, he would be monitored for at least 12 months to check that everything was continuing to move in the right direction.

Yes, following Ben's discharge from CAMHS, a woman came round to our house to talk about how she could help Ben in the transition to university. Ben didn't take to her, and she wasn't much help. But it certainly wasn't what I'd call "monitoring for 12 months".

Far from it.

Yes, Ben is "almost" recovered. But I've been saying "almost" for some time now. The same old loose ends are still loose, flapping around like crazy sometimes. Things like getting back in with his social group, raising his mood, weaning him off calorie counting and weighing food. Plus, of course, the ever-present fear of spiralling out of control and getting fat. I am acutely aware that we need some external help.

During May and June Ben's weight continues to creep up gradually. I'm delighted, of course. But I'm not so sure that Ben agrees.

At first I find myself trying to "justify" the weight gain, like I used to do in the old days when I was terrified of setting off the demon. *What the heck are you doing?* I admonish myself and immediately change tack to: "At this stage you shouldn't be micro-managing your weight; you should have moved on from that."

A bit later Ben (or is it demon?) says: "Would you mind not doing what you did the other day, ever again?"

"Which was what?"

"Looking at my legs in that way."

"What do you mean?"

"When I came in wearing my bathrobe and you looked at my legs 'in that way' as if you were convinced I was skeletal. It's things like this which make it hard for me to trust you."

If it is the demon speaking, then I'd translate it as: "It's things like this which make it hard for me to believe you're not trying to make me fat."

Meanwhile Ben's social life isn't improving. I desperately want him to be out there, with his friends. Sleepovers, cinema trips, meals, parties, band practices, shopping in town or just having a laugh… all those things he used to do before the anorexia whisked him off to Planet Zorg and years of solitary confinement.

How, I wonder, is everything suddenly going to drop into place when he goes away to university? He's missed out on a ton of adolescent social skills. He simply doesn't have them. Having been on his own for nearly three years, in real terms, he has developed other skills. He bosses me around, tells me off and "lectures" me. And the rest of the time he sits in his room either studying or painting his Warhammer models. Or he's downstairs cooking, baking or playing on his computer games. His Facebook page used to have lots of "likes" and comments. Now it's just him posting and me "liking". This is not good - and I have no idea what to do.

The insomnia is back on school days. Which means it may still be here when it comes to the A-level exams, just as it messed up his exams last year. Mind you, messing up A-levels and failing to get into university mightn't be such a bad thing. It would give us another year to push for full recovery on all fronts. It's at times like this that I really miss CAMHS' input. It's now three or four months since Ben was discharged and I know he needs help with getting onto the next rung of the recovery ladder.

The trouble is, almost three years into the anorexia, I have reached burn-out. I just want to rest…

OCCASIONALLY BEN DOES MIX with his friends. Leavers' Day in June is the day when the upper sixth leave to begin their A-level exams. There's a buffet lunch, photographs and usually lots of antics too.

It's the day when, traditionally, everyone dresses in their old school uniform, discarded two years ago after GCSEs. So - like the other families - we've dug out Ben's old green blazer, shirt and tie.

I drop Ben off at school. Everyone's arriving, giggling at the way their friends look like the Incredible Hulk in their skin-tight blazers, the rugby boys' biceps threatening to burst the seams.

There is one exception.

In fact, in his roomy school uniform, Ben could easily be mistaken for a much younger student.

I remember buying this blazer back in Year 9 when Ben began to bulk out into a strapping teenager. I deliberately chose a bigger size with "room to grow". I remember someone's mum talking about how her family went through blazers and shoes like there was no tomorrow because "You wouldn't believe how quickly they shoot up at this age". At £80 a go, I didn't want to have to buy another blazer before Ben reached the uniform-free sixth form.

Initially the blazer was enormous, and Ben hated it.

"Never mind," I said, "You'll grow into it." But, of course, instead of growing into the blazer, Ben did the reverse. By November 2009 it swamped him.

His blazer, sweater, trousers and shirts… they all seemed to get bigger as he got smaller. So I had to buy smaller shirts, trousers and sweaters to avoid him looking ridiculous. But I never bought a new blazer, no matter how massive it looked. I just couldn't afford to.

I was hoping that, two years on, he would have miraculously filled out and the blazer would fit perfectly. But it doesn't. In fact it doesn't look much different from the way it did two years ago. But, then, it always was a huge blazer…

But the big difference is that the boy wearing it today looks much healthier, with a happier expression on his face.

Yet it's still a boy's face and distinctly different from the other sixth formers whose blazers are bursting at the seams with the sleeves half way up their arms.

But, hey, let's celebrate the fact that Ben went into school today - and yesterday too. And he ate with the others at the buffet lunch and took part in the photographs.

This in itself is progress.

I RUN THE IDEA OF FURTHER therapy in front of Ben, to tidy up all the loose ends between now and university.

At first he's not enthusiastic. He insists that it won't help and will be a waste of time. And, as the woman at the private health centre said to me, he has to *want* to have therapy otherwise it won't work. Now, as a legal adult, he has to make the decisions and say yes to therapy. Legally, it can't come from me. So I tell Ben we need to find a way of dealing with the remaining issues, in manageable chunks. Firstly, the period between now and the end of the exams. Secondly, the period between then and the results. And, finally, the period between the results and whatever happens in September - university or no university.

And we need to do this together.

"Together we've done brilliant and amazing things over the past two-and-a-half years," I remind him. "I've become a whiz at finding solutions to problems, no matter how 'hopeless', mainly because I had no choice. Meanwhile you've kept your side of the bargain."

I tell him how proud I am of him. "You've pushed yourself this far," I say. "I didn't do it for you. One day you stood up and refused to let the anorexia eat up any more of your life. You knew the going would be tough, and it has been. But you've refused to give up. You are *still* refusing to give up."

I ask him to have a think about further therapy and we'll talk it through over lunch. He agrees to give it a go.

On Saturday we spend an hour with Amanda, a private dietician specialising in eating disorders. But Ben is cynical. The only clinician he ever really trusted, and he came to trust her implicitly, was Sarah. But I have high hopes that the same will happen with Amanda.

Immediately she introduces the concept that Ben will need to weigh more as he gets older and how men between the ages of 18 and 25 "bulk out" and develop muscle mass naturally. Muscle weighs more than fat. In other words, he won't be "getting fat", he will be building muscle and this is something that will happen naturally.

She also covers a host of other issues that are worrying Ben. Like the concern that, if he doesn't count calories, he may eat "too much" or "too little". And the worry that, if he eats "too much", he "might not be able to stop", will balloon out and become obese.

Amanda points out that, at this stage, it's difficult to say what Ben's set weight as an adult should and will be. It's not an exact science and everyone is different, with a different genetic makeup, skeletal frame and muscle mass - and so on. In other words, one-size-fits-all BMIs aren't helpful when determining the set weight for an individual. Just as I'd always thought.

Thankfully I can tell that Ben is listening. He accepts the science as fact, just as he did with Sarah once his logic and rational thinking returned - the logic that the eating disorder stripped him of for so many months.

Over the next few weeks Ben continues to see Amanda and we see a gradual improvement in his attitude to weight gain. In fact we see a marked improvement all round - eating, mood and socialising. It's all positive stuff, and it seems to be working. I can almost feel the momentum us as Ben begins to move forward again.

29

doing the conga

IT'S JUNE 2012 AND THE FINAL week of the A-level examinations. Ben is anxious and this manifests itself in insomnia again. Worse, he is also resitting some of last year's exams at the same time. I tell him that his exam grades don't matter to us in the slightest.

"But they matter to me," he says. "They matter to my sense of pride. If I mess them up I will feel I have failed."

"But, really, they don't matter at all," I repeat. "If you mess them up then so what? Just re-sit them next year."

"But I really want to go to uni. I want to launch myself back into everything, make a fresh start and begin to live my life again. I couldn't stand having to wait a year."

"You never know," I say thoughtfully. "A year out could be really good for you - as long as you grab it by the horns, do stuff, get out there and so on. It might turn out to be one of the best things you've done. The thing is - uni might be brilliant. I hope it's brilliant. But it's important you don't see it as a 'cure all'. It might not live up to expectations. Or it might take a while to settle in. So another year of sorting stuff out mightn't be a bad idea after all. And, anyway, loads of people take a year out before going to uni."

I make it clear that his dad and I really don't mind what happens. "Be thankful we're not pushy parents," I add with a laugh. "We know you will have done your best under the circumstances - circumstances which are out of your control and not your fault." I have always said to Ben that the most important things for us are his health, happiness and full recovery.

On the final day of exams I take Ben shopping. Thankfully he's smiling when I pick him up from school. Remember the days when I used to dread picking him up? When he'd skulk towards the car as if the world was going to end and give me the silent treatment all the way home? Or yell at me in the voice of the demon?

"The exams were okay," he smiles. "I didn't manage to finish the last essay, and my hand is hurting from writing for three hours, but apart from that - fine."

Excellent, I think, smiling.

We have lunch at Pret, his favourite café. Remember the time when he hid under the stairs noisily sobbing before fleeing into the Saturday shoppers? Purely and simply because he couldn't handle the idea of choosing a sandwich? Today he goes for a huge salad - and it isn't a low calorie one. And he pours French dressing all over it. In the bad old days, the oily French dressing would have remained untouched. Also, in the very bad old days, he wouldn't have been able to choose anything from the menu at all. He would have fled from the restaurant in tears.

Oh, and he also has a bread roll (but sadly without butter) and returns to buy a huge pack of toffee popcorn which he eats as we walk around the shopping mall. In the bad old days he wouldn't have gone for the roll let alone eaten the popcorn so casually. Eating had to be at set times and in a set place, otherwise he couldn't handle it.

In the bad old days I couldn't shop for clothes, shoes, anything. I just didn't have it in me. Today I'm in the shoe shop for an awfully long time looking for some comfortable sandals for our summer vacation. Something I can walk for miles in without getting blisters. Ben gets bored and goes on a wander. Later I find him sitting outside with a large hazelnut Frappuccino. In the bad old days he wouldn't have bought it - period - especially a large one, and even if he had he wouldn't have been able to walk around drinking it in such a relaxed manner. He would have had to sit down in the coffee shop; everything had to be perfect.

Next we pop into Thornton's where he buys some chocolate to replenish his supplies. Remember when Ben used to be drawn to chocolate shops like a magnet? Never to buy, of course, but to "admire" the chocolates as you or I might admire exhibits in a museum - and then admire them for a second or third time, maybe picking up the odd packet with a view to buying before promptly putting it down and fleeing from the shop.

And… and… and… when the assistant asks if he'd like to try a Chocolate Smile he says, "Yes please!" and pops one into his mouth. It's the first time in years that he's said "Yes" to free food samples.

Most important of all, though, is the fact that Ben's been seeing more of his friends. He goes along to an end of exams party at someone's house. I'm thrilled to bits when I pick him up the next day. It's been a great success, albeit aided by some booze.

"The best bit was the psychedelic chill session where I sat with my old friends talking about deep stuff," he says mysteriously. For the first time he actually talked to his friends about his eating disorder, explaining to them why he'd been like he had over the past three years. "Until I got a sudden desire to make toast and marmalade," he says, laughing, followed by an inroad into someone's crumpets at an unearthly hour of the morning before raiding the cupboards to get breakfast. Eating his friend's parents out of house and home? I sincerely hope so!

Crucially, the post-party period is free from guilt or stress. So often in the past what appeared to be a good time would be ruined when Ben returned home. The guilt would come in waves. And before long he would be beating himself up about how much he'd eaten and drunk, convinced he'd been bingeing when he'd simply been eating like a normal teenage boy.

But this time there isn't any of that.

"Oh and by the way, L, Z and K are going to the same uni as me," he says, delighted. "In the same halls of residence."

"Brilliant," I say, mainly because it's evidence of having had a normal conversation with friends rather than hovering on the outside, looking awkward and keeping silent.

Social events feature heavily on Ben's calendar this week. First there's the school Politics trip to London mid-week, followed by W's birthday. Then there's Prize Day on Saturday followed by the Leavers' Ball and - the next day - the Leavers' Chapel Service and Lunch. Then, next week, Ben leaves on a three-day History trip to Poland. A whole week of massive challenges as Ben reminds me when we sit down to do our Contract. These days our Contract has morphed into something we do on an "as needs" basis. But it's still there whenever we need it, just to give Ben that extra bit of encouragement.

Ben rises to the challenge. Prize Day is a success and the Leavers' Ball even more so. And, yes, you're right - that is Ben snaking around the hall with the others doing the Conga, a huge grin on his face. Oh my goodness me… that's him, too, standing on the stage, taking the karaoke microphone to sing Love Train by the O'Jays. Who would have thought it just a few months ago? And, no, he hasn't had too much wine; he's scarcely had any.

SITTING IN BARS EATING ice cream and drinking beer… going back to the hotel, having "deep conversations"… falling asleep, being woken up by J, N and P crashing loudly into the room with some of the girls… being dragged off to the girls' room… some of the boys smoking on the balcony… a furious teacher striding down the corridor wearing nothing but his underpants, knocking on the door and giving them a huge telling off while everyone sniggers… And that was just one night. Ben might have returned a tiny bit lighter due to bad meal planning (not his fault) but, apart from this, the school trip to Poland was… normal!

This, as you can imagine, is music to my ears.

From what I hear, the food in the hotel was inedible. So they went into town and did what normal teenagers normally do: mess around eating this and that, ice creams, pretzels, chocolate, sandwiches… Meanwhile Ben was careful to make sure he was eating enough. He joined the group that went to an Italian restaurant for a proper meal. When they went bowling, Ben grabbed a burger and fries because he knew he had to eat. And Ben, who rarely drinks alcohol, had plenty of beer.

Nevertheless, on his return the scales show a slight weight loss. "It's good in a way," I say encouragingly, "because it shows just how easy it is to lose weight when you're not eating normal meals". I tell him I know it's not his fault, that he'd done his best to eat, even when the others weren't bothering.

But what make me beam from ear to ear is that, throughout these few days in Poland, Ben has been more normal than he's been for years. It is now exactly three years since the anorexia arrived in our lives, during the summer vacation of 2009 - the summer when Ben's exercising and "healthy eating" went extreme and he cut himself off from his friends.

So this trip to Poland makes me happy.

Very happy indeed.

Especially as he quickly, and willingly, puts back the little bit of weight he's lost.

IN AUGUST BEN GETS his exam results. Despite narrowly missing the anticipated A grades he gets his first choice of university, so it's all systems go for September.

I have a set of photographs taken at the party he was invited to on

Results Day - approximately 20 teenagers crowding around a table of drinks in L's garden. Everyone's raising their glass in a "toast". Ben's glass is the highest and there's a huge grin on his face. In another photo he and six of his friends are squashed beside each other on a couple of garden benches, arms around the others' shoulders, drinks at the ready. Ben is in the centre. Looking at them you'd never guess that Ben has been through anorexia. He looks exactly the same as everyone else - and so very, very relaxed and happy. This is Ben, well and truly back in the bosom of his social group. It brings tears to my eyes.

It's not too many weeks ago that I was still anxious about how Ben would cope with being away at university. But I'm astonished at how rapidly he has moved from the last little bit of the woods and out into the brilliant sunshine. He is so normal. In every way. And I have every confidence that, if he continues like this, university will be the making - not breaking - of him.

So, with just two more weeks to go before the 2012 parents dump their offspring off at university, I am just like any other mother: piles of paraphernalia on the spare bed - pots, pans, cleaning stuff, etc, and making the most of the two remaining weeks we have together.

But I already sense Ben is growing up. Already he is becoming independent and putting a natural distance between himself and me, just as any 18 year old or young adult would. After all, why the heck would you want to mix with boring 50-somethings like us when you can have fun with people your own age?

"Another senior moment," he says as my menopausal brain makes me put the breakfast cereal in the fridge.

He is like any other teenage boy taking the mickey out of his parents. And I am certain he will eat properly during the busy university Intro Week - and the following week when everyone gets down to the serious business of studying.

In fact things are going so normally in our household that it's difficult to get used to. A normal mum nagging a normal teenage son about normal things: "Promise me you won't walk home on your own late at night", "Don't forget to put your wallet in a safe place so it doesn't get stolen", "Remember to buy toilet roll and milk", "Don't put the whites in with the darks in the launderette", "Don't drink too much"...

Nag, nag, nag... I imagine I'm just like any other mum in the run up to university. All those little things that you've always done for your child and probably shouldn't - like ironing, sewing on buttons and washing clothes... and always being there to lend them a spare tenner when they run out of cash...

But - yes of course - there are the other issues which are unique to us as a family with a child that's recently been through anorexia. Planning meals that will fit into a chaotic Intro Week... Taking a few frozen meals to see him through those first few evenings... Making sure his luggage is packed with pots, pans and store cupboard staples like tins of tomatoes, rice, pasta, cookies, soup, tuna, cereal, herbs, spices, lentils and other things so he can create a quick meal in minutes. Plus we'll be shopping for fresh stuff like milk, bread, etc. But I guess this, too, is something that "normal" families do on the way to university.

Ben has organised a mentor - a boy from the year above who will be there to look out for him during those first few weeks and months. This boy has a friend with anorexia, so he "gets" the illness more than most, I guess.

There are also accommodation mentors - students from the year above whose job it is to help new students settle into their apartments.

And with a diary jam-packed full of activities from beach parties, BBQs and discos to scuba diving, Buddhist meditation, jazz, radio DJ-ing, ghost walks, pub crawls and treasure hunts, he's bound to meet people he gets on with. Plus, two of his school friends are in the same apartment complex. And the little girl he once insisted he was going to marry… aged just three… is going to be at the other university in the city, just a stone's throw away.

ON FRIDAY EVENING AFTER supper, Ben suddenly appears in the living room armed with brightly wrapped gifts and cards.

"These are to thank you for everything you've done for me over the past 18 years and especially over the past three years," he says as we sit with open mouths.

He's bought us both boxes of chocolates and a card. In it he tells us that he loves us "immensely" and wants to thank us for helping him through his illness as well as nurturing him through his childhood to prepare him to "leave the nest". He says we've prepared him better than any other parents could and that we're the best parents of "all the mums and dads out there". And he thanks us for being there for him when he was "hurt, down or sick" and filling him with the confidence to lead his own life.

And as if that wasn't enough to make us fill up…

…He produces a third card and gift. "These are for you, mum - to thank you for getting me through this."

"But dad helped you get through it too!" I say, not wanting Paul to be left out.

"But you were the one who was with me 24/7 during the dark days. Without your encouragement I mightn't have got through this, let alone be on my way to university on Sunday. I just wanted to thank you especially."

Cue gallons of tears…

In the card he talks about the way we fought the struggle together, not against each other, but against the illness. He talks about my love being a "shining example to the world that love can overcome anything". He talks about the "sheer strength of willpower and motherly love", tells me I am "the most amazing human being I know", above "all other idols in my list of admiration". Finally he thanks me for "being the one that never gave up".

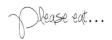

After this I find it hard to concentrate on much else for the remainder of the evening…

OUR LOCAL PIZZA EXPRESS has seen its fair share of ups and downs in the struggle to expel anorexia from Ben's life, and that Sunday evening it sees another episode. This time it's just Paul and me, exhausted from carrying umpteen boxes and bags up two floors into Ben's university apartment. We met the boy in the next room to Ben who seemed very nice. But, apart from him, the apartment was empty.

Paul helped Ben to put up posters while I unpacked all the supermarket shopping into the fridge, freezer and kitchen cupboards. There wasn't much storage space so unfortunately most of the non-perishables had to be stored in Ben's room.

"Ah, this is the life!" I said, sitting on Ben's new bed with my back against the newly postered wall, remembering my days as a student when friends would call into my very similar room for a coffee and we'd sit on the bed talking long into the night.

In Pizza Express, Paul and I order a beer. "I think we need this!" he laughs, ordering an extra-large one for himself. "And let's get some wine, too."

But the atmosphere is subdued. We're both anxious. We can't concentrate on our meal.

I'm well aware that we're not feeling quite as we should. Yes, we should be feeling sadness and loss as our child flies the nest and begins a new chapter in his life, but we should also be feeling a sense of excitement - the same excitement that all three of us had been feeling in the build-up to university.

Yes, it's normal to look at our watches and say wistfully: "I wonder what he's doing now…"

But we're not just wondering; we're worrying.

"He virtually shoved us out of his room earlier," I say, remembering how Ben had commanded us to "Go now!" and when we tried to hug him he snapped "Just go!"

We finish our pizzas in silence, lost in thought.

THE NEXT DAY, IN A BID to stop myself worrying, I decide to blitz Ben's bathroom. I clean and disinfect it from top to bottom, scrubbing, cleaning, polishing, rinsing… I even clean the dusty corners behind the bath which, judging by the filth, haven't been cleaned since the bathroom was installed.

All the time I'm on tenterhooks. I can't relax. I can't stop. I have to keep myself occupied to keep the anxiety at bay.

By the time I go back downstairs to make a late-morning coffee, there's already a message waiting for me on my phone.

30

university challenge

I PLUCK UP THE COURAGE TO click open the message. Ben says he doesn't fit in with the other guys in his apartment and feels lonely… More messages land in my "in box" at lunchtime. I can always tell when all is not well because the first message is always something along the lines of "Hi," and that's all.

Ben feels he isn't ready for university. He feels on a different planet to everyone else and feels way out of his depth socially. His natural instinct, because of the legacy of the anorexia, is to isolate himself rather than putting on a brave face and getting on with it.

I call his mobile. Ben is in floods of tears. He "hates everything". His room feels like a prison cell. He's surrounded by food and cooking utensils because there's no storage in the kitchen. This is triggering the old eating disordered thoughts. Oh, and he feels suicidal.

I spend the next hour or so frantically contacting the various student support services for help. They send a trained counsellor up to his room, but it doesn't make any difference. By the evening Ben is in a terrible state.

"I'll meet you in the Botanical Gardens coffee shop, 10am tomorrow," I tell him. With a heavy heart I sit down and hastily work out a list of options: a Plan A and Plan B.

Plan A is for if he decides to stick it out at university. Plan B is for if the situation is non-salvageable. If possible, we need to avoid a knee-jerk reaction - the urge to flee back to the safety of home.

But I realise this may happen.

With an even heavier heart I drive to Sheffield the next day, parking the car in a road near the Botanical Gardens, close to the student residences.

Ben is standing by the coffee shop looking lost - like a rabbit caught in the headlights. I grab us both a coffee and we find a table in a quiet corner. I get out my notebook and pen, ready to go through the different options.

Ben says he feels way out of his depth. He can't cope. He begins to cry and, as he does, I end up battling back my own tears as we sit opposite each other over our drinks.

I keep calming him down, telling him that this is a "meeting", like our Contract meetings. In other words, it's about sorting things out and about finding workable solutions, just like a business meeting. We can say anything. Indeed we *must* say anything - *everything* in this instance. Nothing must be held back.

"I really thought I was ready for university," he sobs.

"I know you did," I respond, reaching across the table to place my hand over his, fighting back tears of disappointment. University had been such a major focus over the summer, something to look forward to, the chance to start afresh and draw a line under the eating disorder. But when push came to shove, as they say, the reality hit him hard: he simply wasn't ready. Far from it. And on so many counts. Social skills, aversion to the student booze and partying culture, isolation, feeling suicidal and horrendous homesickness… and so on and so forth… and more… The trouble is that none of us realised this until too late.

"I just wanted to show you and dad that I could do it," he whispers, aware that the café is filling up with people who are giving us strange looks. "But I can't…"

"I know you can't, sweetie," I say reassuringly, deciding that Plan

A is a non-starter and Ben is coming home, mainly because at £9,000 a year we can't afford to suck it and see. "But if you leave then you leave with conditions. Okay?"

Yes, okay, he nods.

"Firstly you agree to further therapy to ensure you are ready to try again in 12 months' time." I don't want him to run away and bury his head in the sand, avoiding the issues that still need dealing with. I don't want this to be a backward step. It must be turned into something positive, especially as I instinctively know that Ben will be beating himself up about having "failed" at university.

"Secondly you get a job," I continue. "If you can't get paid work, then you get voluntary work. Thirdly, we work on helping you to become more independent and less reliant on us. Fourthly, we go and see the relevant student support services now. We need to tell them what's going on and talk about the possibility of leaving your place open for 12 months."

Ben readily agrees. It's as if a great weight has been lifted off his shoulders. He begins to calm down.

We finish our coffees and begin the rounds, starting with the accommodation office and ending with student services and the faculty admissions tutors. Everyone sees us immediately. And, without exception, everyone is sympathetic. "You wouldn't believe how many new students we've already seen today!" says the nice lady in student services to reassure Ben. She suggests that Ben gets in touch with her in the spring so she can draw up a special support package should he decide to try again next September. "We'll walk you round the various support services," she says. "And I'm sure we can also walk you through the different accommodation options. You don't have to return to the same apartment block. Or you could commute. Lots of students do." She says that, whatever Ben needs in order to make university a success, they will attempt to provide it.

Ben and I walk back to his apartment feeling much more positive.

We clear his room of as much as I can cram into my car, returning the next day to pick up the rest. I take a last glance at the room where, only a few days before, we were busy putting up posters to make Ben feel at home.

It's been a busy and stressful few days with lots of thinking on my feet. On the motorway I say: "Well done for having the guts to admit that things weren't going right. That takes courage."

I'm as disappointed as hell that it didn't work out. But, deep down, I know we've made the right decision.

A DISMAL BEN GREETS ME the next morning, saying he feels "a failure" and "useless". But I'm ready for this.

Again I remind him that he's been courageous in admitting the problem, rather than letting things spiral downwards. I also say that it takes guts to admit that, yes, there are still issues that need dealing with and which he can't fix by himself, even though over the past few months he really thought he could. And these may need professional help.

As to his gloomy comment that "everyone else" is out there, at university, forging ahead in life, I respond that "everyone else" *isn't* out there, at university. Quite a few of his friends have taken a gap year - and now he is taking a gap year, just like them. And, in three years' time, when "everyone else" has graduated and is busy trying to get a job, Ben will still be at university - *and* he will have valuable work experience behind him. So he'll have a head start. And, hopefully, the UK economy will be in a better place in four years' time. Also, he will be that little bit more mature. Plus, like so many people have said already, taking a gap year is a Good Thing. There are so many Good Reasons to do it.

Onwards and upwards, as they say…

"And let's make this a bloody brilliant year for you, Ben!"

LESS THAN A WEEK LATER, Ben has already set himself a stack of challenges and completed them. He prepares a dazzling CV and drags himself and the CV round dozens of local shops.

He applies for voluntary work, enquires about being a singer in a tribute band and plans a regular Thursday night activity to do with his Warhammer hobby.

Occasionally I throw in the odd suggestion: potential activities he isn't aware of, for example local debating or history groups - and then leave it to him to do the groundwork.

Meanwhile I'm here to offer encouragement and moral support.

Ben returns to the charity shop where he worked over the summer and also - to my surprise and delight - arranges to do two mornings a week as a teaching assistant at his old school.

It's kind of weird getting up early for school again, just like we used to do in the old days.

Except that it couldn't be more different from the old days.

Ben clambers downstairs at the usual time and I can hear him singing at the top of his voice as he prepares a hearty breakfast. On the dot of 7.40am, without any prompting, he climbs into the car and we drive the ten miles to school, listening to the radio and chatting along the way, just like normal people do.

"Have a good day!" I call out as a smiling Ben climbs out of the car and trots off down the alleyway beside the school chapel - the chapel where he was once found hiding, curled in a foetal position, sobbing his heart out.

I pick him up at the end of his shift. The contrast between "then" and "now" strikes me dramatically. Remember the days when I'd be coiled up like a spring, dreading what the demon had in store? The days when Ben would skulk out of the building, dark rings around his eyes, his skull looking out of proportion with his bony body and a deathly expression on his face?

"Had a good morning?" I say casually to the grinning young man that's made his way confidentially across the car park, head held high, dressed in a smart grey suit and tie. "Yes, brilliant," Ben responds, climbing into the car, telling me how the Year 11s hate having to call him "Sir", how it's funny being in the staffroom at break-time and how Sheila, the school nurse, wants him to sing at her leaving "do" in December.

"She's leaving?"

"To work with rescued child soldiers and AIDS orphans in Uganda."

Wow, I think to myself, this woman is incredible. Not for the first time do I muse on how curious it is that Ben's illness should have led us to so many amazing people.

"I'VE BEEN BLOGGING ABOUT it and thought it was time I told you to your face," I tell Ben one morning in mid-October. "I am so very proud of everything you've been doing since you left university. All those conditions we talked about, you've kept to every single one of them - and more. There's no stopping you!"

"I couldn't have done it without you, mum. I mean, if I'd left uni and you'd just sighed and resigned yourself to me wasting my life or something like that..."

"But you haven't wasted your life. You've got out there and got on with things."

"I wouldn't have been able to do it without you..."

"We are a team, you and I," I say hugging him. "A strong team. We work together like a well-oiled machine. But, at the end of the day, it's down to you."

"But I haven't really achieved much, regarding the jobs..."

"That's not your fault. There's a recession on," I remind him. "And don't forget, you're already working four mornings a week doing all that unpaid work."

But, for me, the most amazing thing is how much he's enjoying being at school. No dragging feet, no hiding in the medical centre, no depression, no outbursts, no distressing phone calls or texts. To be honest, if they asked him to work *five* days a week, instead of just two, I believe he'd jump at the prospect. He can't wait to get out of bed and into the classroom to share his encyclopaedic knowledge of history and politics with the sixth formers.

Could this be a career in the making? His former teachers obviously think he has potential, otherwise they wouldn't have agreed to his request. Or they'd have given him "odd jobs" to do like manning the reception desk or whatever. But Ben is standing at the front of the classroom teaching. I mean *really* teaching, while the actual teacher observes. Every time I think about it, my whole being swells with pride. Especially as Ben organised all of this independently, without any prompting or assistance from me.

Who would have thought it?

Who would have thought that, after mourning the end of Ben's school career which ended so negatively after three years of hell, Ben would reinvent himself and embark on a brand new chapter, at the same school?

Ben loves school.

So much so that he's already talking about training to be a teacher once he completes his university degree.

31

trust me, please

BEN IS CONTINUING TO put on weight gradually. Now, to you and me, that's a Good Thing. But unfortunately, even at this late stage, it still isn't Good News to Ben.

"Every time I've got on the scales recently I've put on weight!" the remnants of the demon wail. "How the heck am I supposed to go out and eat meals and stuff when I find I'm putting on weight so fast?"

I've been avoiding the scales for weeks. But, to be honest, I was worried he might be losing again. So I reluctantly agreed to weigh him.

I wish I hadn't.

Damn, why is weight still such a big deal? Should I allow him to cut back so he maintains rather than continues to gain? And possibly risk a downward slide? Bin the scales? And not know whether or not he's losing weight? To be honest, I'd like to see a few more kilos on his frame before we can claim he's "arrived".

Thankfully we've booked a few sessions with an ex-CAMHS psychologist called Joanne who can hopefully fix the remaining glitches.

On Friday morning we meet with her at the now familiar private health centre. Within minutes Joanne gets to the heart of the matter; the elements that remain of the eating disorder - the issues that are preventing Ben from resuming a full and normal life.

There's the way he still feels uncomfortable if he doesn't have his evening meal at a certain time. It's not as rigid as it used to be, but it's still making it difficult to go out in the evening or alter his routine too much. And it got heavily in the way during those few days at university.

Then there's the small issue of Ben thinking about food pretty much all of the time, over and above most other things. Also the way he worries about putting on weight. "I have a wardrobe of clothes I can't get into," he complains to Joanne.

"Also, when I went out for a run the other day someone shouted 'Run fat boy run!'. Why would they do that if I wasn't putting on weight? I think about food all the time. I want to eat all the time and then I feel greedy."

I notice he uses the word "greedy" a few times.

Ben is still worried that his weight will spiral out of control. Yet at the same time he's worried that if he cuts back on food it will do the opposite and he could be dragged back down into the eating disorder. "So I feel as if I'm between a rock and a hard place," he protests.

"Can you tell in advance if you've put on a kilo?" Joanne asks.

"Oh yes. And I feel cr*p. I have a naturally big frame, you see, and so a little bit of weight makes me look far bigger than I actually am. I also have a round face which looks worse if I put on a bit of weight. When I was a few kilos lighter my features were much sharper and I preferred that."

Hmn, I can see Joanne thinking. "Do you think I would be able to notice if you put on a kilo?" she asks followed by: "What we need to do is to work on getting you from 'here' to 'there', from where you are now in terms of rigid thinking, food and weight worries to a position where you don't worry and are sufficiently free of anxiety and restrictions to allow you to resume the kind of life you want to lead - and the kind of life you would *need* to lead in order to have a successful life at university."

She explains that she doesn't expect the changes to happen overnight; they need to be achieved in small manageable steps.

"Although you might think you haven't come very far over the past few months and feel in a bit of a rut, I suspect that if you compared where you are now with where you were then you would see quite a dramatic change. And you are already doing so many positive things, like the voluntary work and so on."

I nod my head in agreement.

Don't get me wrong, these aren't massive sticking points. Not massive when you compare them to the enormous issues we've had to overcome in the past.

We are in a very different place these days, a much better place. It's just that I am aware that there are still several sticking points - issues that still need ironing out before Ben can resume a normal anorexia-free life again.

The trouble is that Ben suddenly decides that he no longer wants formal therapy. He can fix things himself. So, after a couple more sessions with Joanne, we call it a day. As the old adage goes: "You can lead a horse to water, but you can't make it drink."

But if the "horse" is managing to get its liquids from elsewhere, then maybe, at this late stage, it's okay to let him see how it goes.

GETTING YOUR CHILD THROUGH an eating disorder is damn tough, we all know this. But what happens when they reach their target weight?

What no-one ever told me is how your child is supposed to come to terms with this. Their weight is okay, but obviously it's been going up for some time. What if it continues to go up? What if it never stops? What if he begins to blob out and get fat? These are the kind of fears that are spinning around Ben's head at this stage.

CAMHS always said: "Don't worry; we'll never let your weight spiral out of control once you reach your target weight."

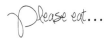

That's fine, in principle.

The trouble is, when this finally happened - or at least when Ben reached a weight that fell safely within the healthy boundaries - CAMHS were no longer around.

I've heard it said that full recovery is all about getting to a stage where this kind of thinking no longer bothers you. Food begins to take its normal place in everyday life rather than dominating it. Gaining the odd extra kilo or two is no longer a worry. But what "they" never said is how you get from where Ben is *now:* a safe weight but extremely anxious about continuing to put on weight - to where he *should be:* fully weight restored and content.

Or, I think to myself, maybe some people take years to reach this point? Not because they're not "fully recovered" as such, but because this is the kind of person they are.

All I know is that, despite some recent ups and (some quite distressing but thankfully temporary) downs, Ben is continuing to push himself in the right direction. Now and again, the anorexia thoughts lurk in the background, which is why he still asks if we can "do points" to help him deal with challenges.

There is also the issue of socialising, which hasn't really improved. Especially since most of his friends are now at university or on gap year projects.

On the other hand, he has no issues with going into school or socialising with his Warhammer crowd down at Games Workshop. So, to be truthful, it looks as if he's dealing with this too.

In his own way. Just like normal 19 year olds do.

And, if the general trend is positive, then Ben's "own way" is okay as far as I'm concerned.

But, of course, I'll be keeping a discreet eye on progress.

SHORTLY BEFORE CHRISTMAS the amazing and awesome

Sheila, the school nurse, says her goodbyes. The school hall is packed with people wishing her well in her new vocation as a nurse working with rescued child soldiers and AIDS orphans in Uganda.

It's clear that there are scores of other families that she's supported, just as she's supported us. And the funny thing is, I suspect that each family feels they were the "only family". That was one of the many unique things about Sheila; she made everyone feel special. Unlike many clinicians, she never kept a "professional distance" where genuine love, humanity and compassion were needed. She is loved by hundreds of people.

One mother stands at the front of the hall, talking about the way Sheila supported her family when her daughter developed a serious heart condition.

Just as with Ben, Sheila opened the medical centre as a bolt-hole where this girl could escape from the kids who were bullying her about her illness.

"I can't describe what it's like to hold your unconscious daughter in your arms and see her turn blue in front of you," the mother says, choking back the tears, describing one of the lowest points in her daughter's illness.

It was Sheila who helped her come to terms with the illness, who encouraged her to pick herself up, dust herself down and do what needed to be done. In other words, to find the courage and strength to face the illness and deal with it as best she could - and guide her daughter towards recovery. And Sheila was always there, at the end of the phone, email or text, or in person, to provide extra support and advice - or simply a shoulder to cry on.

It all sounds so familiar.

Like the time Sheila invited me round to her house for a meal. And the other time she took me out for lunch - on her - so I could update her on Ben's progress. She didn't have to do that. It wasn't part of her job description. But she did it. And I suspect she did it for many other people, too.

"Sheila's house is like an 'open house'," says the next well-wisher who's come to the front of the hall to speak. "It's permanently jam-packed full of people. Friends, neighbours, people from church, former school pupils and families…"

"Big hug!" I say as we leave, giving Sheila a massive bear hug and wishing her all the best for the future. "I can't thank you enough for everything you've done for us."

She asks about this book. After all, it was she who suggested I write it in the first place.

"I've got a printed proof," I say. "But I want to re-write some of it. Parts of it just don't get across exactly how bad things were - or how good they were once things improved. I'll be doing some more work on it in the new year." I promise to mail her a copy when it's finally published.

Why has Sheila decided to leave everything - a comfortable house, lovely job, good income, friends and family - for an unpaid job in a village in Northern Uganda? ("I've insisted on a sit-down toilet," she said earlier this evening. "And a big table where I can sit down and talk to people.")

"It was one of the boys in this photo," she explains, pointing at the PowerPoint slideshow. "He'd seen both his parents killed in front of his eyes and would sit there silently, blank eyes, no emotion. And he'd shrink from human contact." Last summer, when Sheila was working as a volunteer during the school summer holidays, she gradually began to get through to this boy. It wasn't until the penultimate day of her stay that she finally got a result.

"We took the boys swimming," she says. "I decided to place a towel around his shoulders. He didn't need a towel of course; out there it's so hot you just dry naturally, but I thought, hey, I'll do this and see what happens. Almost immediately he pulled the towel around his shoulders and nudged himself over to me for a cuddle.

Probably his first warm human contact since his parents were killed. Suddenly I realised that you can't just dip in and out of this sort of thing. You can't just go for eight weeks or whatever, do some good and then fly back to your cosy home and career. By coming home I was breaking that precious new bond and I found this difficult to deal with." That was when Sheila decided she had to do this full time.

So she handed in her notice at school.

What a woman.

What on earth would we have done without her?

DESPITE THE UPS AND DOWNS, things seem to be going relatively okay in the lead up to Christmas 2012. During the "down times" it's almost as if Ben is letting off steam. He always feels a heck of a lot better afterwards. Paul and I don't necessarily feel better, especially following a particularly distressing "blip" in mid-December. But if Ben feels okay, and these are just "blips" and not a relapse, then that's all that matters.

As I always said, when Ben is walking around the house singing at the top of his voice then all is right with the world. And he sings a lot these days. Especially on school days.

"Thank you for sharing your emotions and thoughts with me recently," I say to him one afternoon as we do our Contract which, these days, is really only used as an opportunity to chat about progress. "Telling me you felt really down the other weekend couldn't have been easy. But, as I am sure you can see, it's the only way I can know what's going on in your head and try to help you. So, thank you, I really appreciate it."

I tell him that, ultimately, he is at the helm of his recovery and I am just here to support him when - or if - he needs it.

We have some really good conversations. Really positive. Which is why, despite the recent dips, I am convinced that everything is going in the right direction.

Of course we don't talk about the eating disorder all the time. In fact we talk about it less and less, most of the time only when Ben asks if we can "do points". He sees the anorexia as something dark and repugnant, memories he'd rather forget. To him, the anorexia is past tense and he wants to move on. Yes, Ben gets angry and depressed at the way he lost three years of his adolescence to this illness and, yes, there are still a few remnants of the eating disorder that remain, but Ben is dealing with these in his own way. Slowly but surely, just as he's managed to deal with everything else. And let's face it, since turning a corner in October 2010, he's managed to deal with a heck of a lot. Successfully.

"What about university?" I ask him one day. "Do you think you'll be ready to try again this September?"

"I don't know," he says, "I'm still thinking about it. I'll let you know nearer Easter."

But at least he is looking forward to the future.

And whenever I put on my negative hat and begin to panic over some recent "blip" he'll say: "You don't honestly think I want to give in to the ED thoughts? I loathe the legacy of ED as much as you do. Trust me, please… Trust that I'm getting myself through this. Just stop fretting."

And I must. I know I must.

32

happy ever after?

LAST SUMMER I'D ALMOST completed this book. I'd read it through umpteen times and sent off chunks to people to proof-read. I'd also read it aloud to Ben, page by page, while he made his own comments and observations which have been incorporated into the pages.

Back in the summer it really did feel as if we'd reached the end of a massive chapter in our lives and were moving on. Ben was relaxed, happy, confident, mixing with his friends and excited about the prospect of university. I felt as if we'd finally left the eating disorder and its legacy behind.

So, six months on, how do I feel?

Recovery from anorexia is never going to be a straight path. You go up and down, round and round, take wrong turns, go several steps back, wind up in a dead-end, then get stuck in deep mud for a while. Then you begin to move forward again.

The offer of further therapy is still open if he feels he ever needs it. But, at present, Ben is happy working on the outstanding issues himself. "To be honest, mum, I used to come away from therapy sessions feeling worse than when I went in," he says. He insists that all the therapists seem to do is resurrect old demons, going back over things he'd prefer to forget.

He says he wants to move on.

"Fine," I reply. "As long as we get to see visible, lasting results."

And hopefully his strong will and determination are what will ensure the remnants of the eating disorder eventually fade away for good.

In the meantime, Paul and I are keeping a discreet eye on him - from a distance. Like any parent of a child who has come through a serious illness and where there are still a number of outstanding issues, there will always be the worry that the anorexia could come back. Relapses happen. And we will fight tooth and nail to ensure that the anorexia demon never, ever takes over our son again, whatever his age.

Last night Ben cooked dinner: roast beef with a peppercorn crust, red wine and onion gravy, roast potatoes and vegetables. We all sat around the dinner table and tucked in. Ben had seconds followed by a homemade sticky toffee pudding with ice cream and further snacks throughout the evening.

Just now, Ben popped into my office where I'm tapping away on the keyboard and announced that the chilli chocolate Paul's been handing round is "yummy" and if I didn't want mine then he'd have it. Personally, I'm not a big fan of chilli and chocolate as a combo, so I was glad to hand it over.

"Oh and you're going to love my chockywocky triangles," he added, munching away on the latest mouth-watering delight to emerge from our kitchen. Unlike the summer of 2009, I can depend on him to tuck into everything he bakes. *And* to add golden syrup, ice cream or - in the case of his delicious carrot cake muffins the other day - vanilla buttercream frosting.

Looking back, there's no doubt that 2012 was a year of ups and downs, of challenges and of glitches. Ben's mood and motivation went up and down as he reached a number of frustrating plateaux and stumbling blocks. But it was also a year of tremendous successes and emotional highs. It was the year that Ben sat his A-levels, won his place at university and prepared to leave home. It was the year he subsequently decided that, no, he wasn't ready for university and needed time to think. It was the year when he morphed from school student to teaching assistant - yet another unexpected twist in a year packed with surprises.

Crucially, 2012 was a year when we could see the light shining brightly at the end of the tunnel, a light that had seemed so dim and unattainable in past years. Sometimes the light seemed so close we could almost touch it. Yet at other times it seemed to be moving further away. Then, in January 2013, the light began to shine brightly again.

Just like the weather there will be sunny days and cloudy days. And doubtless there will be downright stormy days. But everyone has days like these; it's a normal part of life.

I suspect this is what recovery from anorexia is like. There is never going to be a clear-cut moment when you can say, hand on heart, that "Yesterday my child had anorexia. Today he or she is completely recovered". Eating disorders aren't like illnesses where you can take a course of medication and know that, in a short while, you'll be as right as rain. If only…

And I also suspect that, having lived with this thing for so long, there are elements of today's Ben that are now an integral part of his personality, part of who he is.

In other words, he will never be the same Ben that he was before the eating disorder. He's been through hell and high water. He's experienced - and had the strength and courage to overcome - challenges that most teenagers will never have to go through. And, when you've been through a serious illness, it's bound to change you. Some of these changes are good, others not so good. And there will always be dark memories which will hopefully fade with time.

But we are all confident that the worst of the anorexia is long gone. The "demon", the rages, the numbness, the deep depression, the violence, the hopelessness… The resistance to eating, the fear of fatty foods, the hurtling downhill unable to stop… The protruding bones, the sores from over-exercising, the compulsion to relentlessly exercise from morning to night, the scary pulse rate, the fear of "sitting around all day doing nothing", the angry dry skin… And those blank eyes that will haunt me forever. Almost as much as the voice I came to dread above everything else: the deep, slow monotone… the voice of the "anorexia demon". Like when you play a 78rpm record at 33rpm.

All of these are gone. This in itself brings a happy ending to our story.

Perhaps, in a second edition of this book, I will add an *Epilogue* about how the remnants of the eating disorder eventually disappear. The fear of getting fat, of spiralling out of control, the calorie counting and weighing food, the social anxiety…

And I would love to think that, yes, Ben can deal with these issues by himself, without any outside help.

We've already set a new, higher weight target which I'd like him to reach over the next week or so. And Ben has accepted that, yes, his weight will increase as he gets older. Plus, as you would expect with any normal person, the scales go up and they go down. But it's nothing that can't be easily fixed by a few extra hundred calories a day for a while.

Ben is gradually discovering that he won't suddenly "spiral out of control" and get obese. He still finds it hard to come to terms with gaining a few extra kilos permanently, but we're working on it.

In a few months' time he'll need to decide whether or not he's ready for another attempt at university in September. What do Paul and I think? To be honest, we're not sure. Another year off wouldn't be a bad thing. But, at the end of the day, it's Ben's decision.

All we want is for Ben to be healthy and happy.

All the other things in life can wait.

So, for now, all I can say is *watch this space…*

acknowledgments

THANK YOU TO EVERYONE who has supported us in our battle with anorexia. The following is in no particular order…

Firstly thank you to the CAMHS team for providing 24 months of support. Thank you to Sheila, the school nurse, who took Ben - and me - under her wing and suggested I put our experiences into a book. I wish you all the best in your new vocation in Uganda; I know you will be awesome. Also, thank you to the Headmaster and staff for going out of their way to help in any way they could.

I must thank my husband Paul for being my rock through the dark days. At times the going was tough but you were always there for me. Thank you to my sister for being there on those Sunday afternoons when I needed a shoulder to cry on and the hundreds of other times you supported Paul, Ben and me. Thank you to my parents. Dad, I'm so sorry you passed away before you could see your grandson fully recover.

Thank you to all the FEAST-ies from the *Around the Dinner Table* forum and my Facebook friends. You know who you are! Thank you to my fabulous volunteer proof-readers and the other people that offered to read through my book and provide me with great reviews. Thank you, also, to Oxford University's Health Experiences Research Group for permitting me to use some quotes from Ulla's interview with Ben.

Finally words can't express how thankful I am to Sue - the tiny woman with the big smile and even bigger heart who supported me, selflessly, until her illness took her away.

And, of course, thank you once again to my wonderful son, Ben, for being courageous enough to allow me to share his story with you.

by the same author

Anorexia Boy Recovery: a mother's blog about her teenage son's recovery from anorexia, Part I (2011) - by Bev Mattocks

Anorexia Boy Recovery: a mother's blog about her teenage son's recovery from anorexia, Part II (2012) - by Bev Mattocks

Interested in reading our story in more detail? Since January 2011 I've been writing a regular blog about my teenage son's recovery from anorexia: ***AnorexiaBoyRecovery.blogspot.co.uk***.

I love blogs. As a serial journal writer I've been doing this kind of writing since… well… for an awful long time: first my teenage journals, then a regular blog for a regional newspaper and blogs for various business clients - and now this blog.

I love it when someone tells me how much my blog has helped them in their own family's battle with anorexia. Of course I'm neither a clinician nor an expert; I am just an ordinary mum. But when you suddenly find yourself on this devastating journey, it can be reassuring to know that others have been along this road too. To know what they went through, to know what signs to watch out for and to know what worked. And, importantly, during those many false summits and disappointments, to know how they found the strength to carry on fighting and guide their child towards recovery. This is why I write my blog.

But, because blogs are difficult to scroll through or refer back to, I made the decision to publish my blog in paperback: in two parts - 2011 and 2012 - both of which are available on Amazon and as ebooks.

Like my blog, these 300+ page books describe our battle with anorexia in more detail, including countless incidents that haven't been included in *Please eat* in order to compress the story line and keep the book to a manageable length.

So, if you're interested in reading more about our long battle with anorexia, these books are definitely well worth a read. And, to keep up to date with Ben's progress in 2013 and beyond, why not follow my blog?

Best wishes,

Bev Mattocks, February 2013

resources

Websites

www.aroundthedinnertable.org - The *Around the Dinner Table* forum provides support for parents and caregivers of anorexia, bulimia and other eating disorder patients

www.feast-ed.org - *FEAST (Families Empowered and Supporting Treatment of Eating Disorders)* is an international organisation of, and for, parents to help loved ones recover from eating disorders by providing information and mutual support, promoting evidence-based treatment, and advocating for research and education

www.b-eat.co.uk - *BEAT* provides helplines, online support and a network of UK-wide self-help groups to help adults and young people in the UK beat their eating disorders

www.mengetedstoo.co.uk - *Men Get Eating Disorders Too* is a UK based charity dedicated to representing and supporting the needs of men with eating disorders

www.maudsleyparents.org - *Maudsley Parents* is a US based volunteer organisation of parents who have helped their children recover from anorexia and bulimia through the use of a family-based treatment known as the Maudsley approach, an evidence-based therapy for eating disorders

www.anorexiabulimiacare.org.uk - *ABC* is a UK national eating disorder organisation that support sufferers and their family and friends towards full recovery from eating disorders.

www.kartiniclinic.com - the *Kartini Clinic* is a US based medical and mental health treatment facility dedicated exclusively to the treatment of eating disorders in children and young adults - this website includes a stack of useful information, videos, etc

www.drsarahravin.com - *Dr Sarah Ravin* is a US based eating disorders therapist whose website includes a highly informative blog plus other useful information

www.anorexiaboy.co.uk - my website which talks about our fight to help our son recover from anorexia

www.youtube.com/user/CandMedPRODUCTIONS/videos - C&M Productions' eating disorder resource for carers promoting evidenced based treatment and hope

www.thenewmaudsleyapproach.co.uk - an excellent resource for professionals and carers of people with eating disorders

http://eatingdisorders.ucsd.edu - *University of California, San Diego, Eating Disorders Center for Treatment and Research*

www.youthhealthtalk.org/young_people_Eating_disorders - a project by the *Health Experiences Research Group at the University of Oxford* where young people talk about their experiences of living with, and recovering from, an eating disorder.

www.youngminds.org.uk - *Young Minds* is the UK's leading charity committed to improving the emotional wellbeing and mental health of children and young people.

Books

Skills-based Learning for Caring for a Loved One with an Eating Disorder: The New Maudsley Method - by Janet Treasure

Help Your Teenager Beat an Eating Disorder - by James Lock and Daniel Le Grange

Treating Bulimia in Adolescents: A family-based approach - by James Lock and Daniel Le Grange

Decoding Anorexia: How Breakthroughs in Science Offer Hope for Eating Disorders - by Carrie Arnold

Brave Girl Eating: The inspirational true story of one family's battle with anorexia - by Harriet Brown

Just Tell Her to Stop: family stories of eating disorders - by Becky Henry, Founder of Hope Network, LLC

Eating With Your Anorexic - by Laura Collins
Running on Empty: A Diary of Anorexia and Recovery - by Carrie Arnold
A Girl Called Tim: Escape from an Eating Disorder Hell - by June Alexander
Boys Get Anorexia Too - by Jenny Langley
Hope with Eating Disorders: a self-help guide for parents, carers and friends of sufferers - by Lynn Crilly
My Kid is Back - by June Alexander

Blogs

anorexiaboyrecovery.blogspot.co.uk - the blog which I began writing in January 2011
ed-bites.blogspot.co.uk - a super blog by Carrie Arnold, author and recovered former anorexia sufferer
www.laurassoapbox.net - a fabulous blog by Laura Collins, founder of FEAST and ATDT
charlotteschuntering.blogspot.co.uk - a blog by Charlotte, one of the ATDT members
http://hopenetwork.info/beckys-blog - a blog by Becky Henry, Founder of Hope Network, LLC
onemoremum.wordpress.com – a mother's blog about life with her teenage daughter who is recovering from anorexia

18015101R00142

Made in the USA
Charleston, SC
11 March 2013